Alaba O. Ojo
C. N Anigbogu

Petroleum Products Altered Cardiovascular Function, PCV & Plasma Lipid

AF138605

Alaba O. Ojo
C. N Anigbogu

Petroleum Products Altered Cardiovascular Function, PCV & Plasma Lipid

Effects Of Petroleum Products And Their Water Soluble Fractions On Cardiovascular Function, PCV And Plasma Lipid In Rats

LAP LAMBERT Academic Publishing

Impressum / Imprint

Bibliografische Information der Deutschen Nationalbibliothek: Die Deutsche Nationalbibliothek verzeichnet diese Publikation in der Deutschen Nationalbibliografie; detaillierte bibliografische Daten sind im Internet über http://dnb.d-nb.de abrufbar.

Alle in diesem Buch genannten Marken und Produktnamen unterliegen warenzeichen-, marken- oder patentrechtlichem Schutz bzw. sind Warenzeichen oder eingetragene Warenzeichen der jeweiligen Inhaber. Die Wiedergabe von Marken, Produktnamen, Gebrauchsnamen, Handelsnamen, Warenbezeichnungen u.s.w. in diesem Werk berechtigt auch ohne besondere Kennzeichnung nicht zu der Annahme, dass solche Namen im Sinne der Warenzeichen- und Markenschutzgesetzgebung als frei zu betrachten wären und daher von jedermann benutzt werden dürften.

Bibliographic information published by the Deutsche Nationalbibliothek: The Deutsche Nationalbibliothek lists this publication in the Deutsche Nationalbibliografie; detailed bibliographic data are available in the Internet at http://dnb.d-nb.de.

Any brand names and product names mentioned in this book are subject to trademark, brand or patent protection and are trademarks or registered trademarks of their respective holders. The use of brand names, product names, common names, trade names, product descriptions etc. even without a particular marking in this work is in no way to be construed to mean that such names may be regarded as unrestricted in respect of trademark and brand protection legislation and could thus be used by anyone.

Coverbild / Cover image: www.ingimage.com

Verlag / Publisher:
LAP LAMBERT Academic Publishing
ist ein Imprint der / is a trademark of
OmniScriptum GmbH & Co. KG
Heinrich-Böcking-Str. 6-8, 66121 Saarbrücken, Deutschland / Germany
Email: info@lap-publishing.com

Herstellung: siehe letzte Seite /
Printed at: see last page
ISBN: 978-3-659-76885-9

Zugl. / Approved by: Lagos, University of Lagos, Dissertation, 2007

DEDICATION

This work is dedicated to the almighty God for His Faithfulness.

ACKNOWLEDGEMENT

Unreserved appreciation goes to almighty God. I acknowledge the effort of my supervisor, Dr. C. N. Anigbogu, for his encouragement, guidance, sense of direction and challenges which made me achieve what I thought impossible. My appreciation goes to all lecturers, at the Department of Physiology, University of Lagos for their dedication towards producing vibrant physiologist, my thanks also goes to the Chief Technologist, Mr. S.A. Adesina and his assistant, Mrs. Olubunmi. I appreciate the encouragement I got from friends and colleagues, the support of ; my siblings, parent and wife who are looking towards seeing me at the peak of my career. The report of International Programme on chemical safety (1982) Committee; criteria 20,selected petroleum products, set up by World Health Organization gave insight to parts of the review in this work.

TABLE OF CONTENT

LIST OF TABLES

LIST OF FIGURES

CHAPTER ONE
1.1 INTRODUCTION

Petroleum exploration and exploitation are the mainstay of Nigeria's economy. One drastic effect associated with these is the contamination of the immediate environment (terrestrial, aquatic and arboreal habitat) with hydrocarbons (Amadi *et al.*, 1993). Most of the lands in the oil producing areas in Nigeria are under cultivation because the people depends on farming and fishing for their survival, hydrocarbon eventually gets into man and animal through ingestion of contaminated food and water or bio-concentration through food chain (Egborge, 1991). Occupational exposure to petroleum products due to volatility of certain components causes inhalation hazard in the refineries and other industries where petroleum products are used as raw materials in processing other finished products. Achuba and Osakwe,(2004) reported that presence of hydrocarbon in the body system induces oxidative stress through generation of free radicals. These free radicals causes lipid per-oxidation that damages critical cellular macromolecules like DNA, lipids, protein and inactivation of antioxidant enzymes (Achuba, 2005). The toxic effects of petroleum hydrocarbons are exerted on various organs of living systems such as the lung, liver and kidney. But much work has not been done on the effects of hydrocarbons on cardiovascular system.

Groundwater contamination due to petroleum pipeline corrosion, rupture and/or vandalism in urban and rural areas is not uncommon. Many household chemicals and agricultural chemicals are made of petroleum products. Thus the majority of the population are exposed directly or indirectly to petroleum products whose route of contact could be through inhalation, dermal or accidental ingestion (Jessup and Leighton, 1996).

Hydrocarbons are highly lipophilic and are easily absorbed through inhalation, dermal exposure or ingestion. The volume of distribution in the body systems has been shown to be dependent on the proportion of lipid content of each organ until saturation occurs (Gerarde, 1963; Bohlen *et al.*, 1997). Epidermal hypertrophy, hyper-plasia, hyper-keratosis and depilation as well as erythema has been documented after dermal application of hydrocarbons. Hydrocarbons have also been found to have narcotic effect and cause central nervous system depression after chronic inhalation in rats (Hoekstra and Philips, 1963). Aspiration of kerosene into lung causes pulmonary oedema and haemorrhages (Gerarde, 1959). Berepubo *et al.*, (1994), reported that short exposure to crude oil led to inhibition of growth in weaned rabbit.

Dede and Kaglo, (2001), have shown that some fishes accumulate and store aromatic hydrocarbon from oil spillage and pass them to higher trophic level, even several years later. The ingestion of crude petroleum contaminated diet imposed a reciprocal relationship between HDL- cholesterol and LDL- cholesterol in the plasma of rabbit and reduced blood glucose (Achuba, 2005; Ben-David *et al.*, 2001). Uncontrolled exposure to petroleum additives like tetraethyl lead (iv) have been revealed to have negative impact on lipid metabolism, (Ademuyiwa, *et al.*, 2005)

Renal insufficiency has been associated with abnormalities in lipoprotein metabolism in both early and the advanced stages of chronic renal failure; these include alterations in apo-lipoproteins A and B, high density lipoproteins and triglycerides (Crook *et al.*, 2003). Epidemiological studies have revealed that hypertension and type 2 diabetes tend to occur together as part of a syndrome of metabolic abnormalities that includes insulin resistance, raised plasma triglyceride and low high density lipoprotein (HDL) cholesterol level, (Al- Malroos, *et al.*, 2001). Aitman *et al*, (1997), suggested after epidemiological survey, that diabetes might be associated with an underlying metabolic disturbance in certain population in which raised plasma cholesterol levels are accompanied with insulin resistances.

A large body of evidence, including work on animal models and clinical trials, has established that plasma lipids play role in atherosclerotic cardiovascular disease, which begin with angina pectoris at early stage; as a result of endothelia damage and loss of physiological vasomotor activities caused by dyslipdemia, (ICEP, 1993). A dysfunctional endothelium, will impair the expression of endothelins and endothelin A and B receptors as well as Nitric oxide production and activity. Consequently, response to changes in intravascular conditions to constrict and dilate is affected, this can cause hypertension (Ruben, *et al.*, 2006).

The main objectives of this study are to investigate effects of some petroleum products and their water soluble fractions(WSF) on plasma lipid profile and cardiovascular function in experimental rats.

1.2 LITERATURE REVIEW
1.2.1CLASSIFICATION
a. CRUDE OIL

Crude oil are essentially very complex mixture of many thousands of different hydrocarbons originated from the decomposition and transformation of aquatic, mainly marine animals and plants that became buried under successive layers of mud and silt some 15-500 millions years ago. Depending on the source, the oils contain various proportions of straight and branched paraffin, cyclo-paraffins and naphthenic, aromatic, and polynuclear aromatic hydrocarbons (IPCS, 1982). In crude oil, gaseous and solid compounds occur dissolved in liquid fraction. As a general rule, under normal conditions of temperature and pressure, up to 4 carbon atoms are gaseous, those with 5-20 carbon atoms are liquid and those above 20 carbons exist as solid (IPCS, 1982).

The sulfur contents of crude oil ranges from less than 2 to 60g/kg, Nitrogen from 19 to 20g/kg, the sulfur exists as sulfide, mercaptan, thiophenes and more complex organic compounds while Nitrogen compounds exist as complex and mostly unidentified structures. Crude oil also contain naphthenic acids and phenolic compound (petroleum handbook, 1966). Crude oil contains mostly, if not all known elements, mainly in few small quantities except nickel, molybdenum and mercury that sometime could be up to 10mg/kg and vanadium 50mg/kg (Mason, 1966).

Appearance and consistency ranges from yellowish brown mobile liquids to black viscous semi-solid due to different proportions of various molecular types and sizes of hydrocarbon (IPCS, 1982). They are usually classified into three groups accordingly; paraffin base crude oil- contain paraffin wax but little or no asphaltic matter, asphaltic based crude oil- which contain large proportion of asphaltic matter with little or no paraffins and mixed crude oil-which contains paraffin wax and asphaltic matter along with naphthene with certain proportions of aromatic hydrocarbon, (petroleum Hand book, 1966).

b. PETROLEUM SOLVENTS

These represent the intermediate refinery stream from which they are distilled, it is a complex mixture of hydrocarbons reflecting the constituent of crude oil. Due to high degree of over-lapping of the constituents, it can only by classified based on distillation range:

Special- Boiling point solvents (SPPS). These are highly refined naphtha fraction with specially selected boiling ranges which may be narrow or wide but fall within limits of 30- 160^{0}C. consumer products in this range include petroleum ether lighter fluid, spot remover and rubber solvent. They are classified according to boiling ranges e.g. 62/82 (IPCS, 1982). SBPS contain hydrocarbon mixture between C-5 to C-9; normal and branched paraffins, cyclo-paraffins and aromatic compounds with traces of olefins.

White spirits – this contain mixture of hydrocarbon between C-7 and C-12 with boiling rages of 150-220^{0}C. they are classified into low aromatic grade which contain 15-20% aromatic hydrocarbon and high aromatic grade which contain about 45% aromatic hydrocarbon, other constituent include normal and branched paraffins as well as cyclo-paraffins (naphthanic hydrocarbon) and traces of olefins. This range fall between gasoline and kerosene, examples include: stoddard solvent, mineral spirits, low aromatic white spirits (LAwS) and turpentine substitute (IPCS, 1982).

High boiling aromatic solvents. This group include solvents with aromatic content of 50-100% with boiling range of 160-300^{0}C, it consists of mixture of hydrocarbons, above C-9. They are highly purified "white solvents which could exist mainly in crude oils or during secondary processing like thermal or catalytic processing (Petroleum hand book, 1966).

c. LUBRICATING BASE OILS AND RELATED OILS, GREASES AND WAXES

These are limited group of petroleum products in the boiling range of 300-700^{0}C derived from high-vacuum distillation of the crude distilling process, they under further refining before being used. Related oils products are produced by blending of base oils to obtained desired physical properties along with small amount of chemicals additives. Base oils are characterized base on viscosity and viscosity index; the higher the viscosity index the less the change in viscosity with temperature low viscosity index (LVI) medium viscosity index (MIVI) and high viscosity index (HVI). (IPCS 1982).

Base oil, are very complex mixture of hundreds to thousand of different hydrocarbons in the range of C-17 and higher, examples include white oils, medicinal

9

oil, technical white oils, aromatic extracts petroleum waxes and microcrystalline wax (IPCS 1982).

d. BITUMEN
This is the solid and semi solid residue obtained from distillation of crude oil and it also exists as natural deposit, it range from black to dark brown in colour, and also from a highly viscous liquid to solid and brittle substance at normal ambient temperature, constituents varies with source and process of manufacture. Mixture of six samples was found to contain, 32% asphalt, 32% resins, 14% saturated hydrocarbon and 22% aromatic hydrocarbons. (Simmers, 1964; IPCS, 1982).

1.2.2 SOURCES
a. NATURAL SOURCES
Crude oils are purely natural products, they are produced from artificial well, natural seepage occur in various part of the world. Other petroleum products are components of crude oils (IPCS, 1982).

b. MAN MADE SOURCES AND USES
World production of crude oil in 1973 was about 2,900 million tones and over 3,200 million in 1979. The estimate of production of petroleum solvents in 1979 is 9 million tones. The production rate of petroleum products is increasing every year so also the rate of exposure (IPCS, 1982). Crude oils are used as fuel, road construction and malaria control. Petroleum solvents are used as solvents, thinner in lacquers and paints, lighter fuels, pesticides, plastic and rubber, extraction solvents; for perfume, vegetable oils, oil and fat of animal origin, e.t.c. (IPCS, 1982).

Base oils and lubricating oils are used in various way by entire population as lubricating oil, textile oil, process oil, medicinal white oil, among others, and those oils sometime contain carcinogenic nitrosamines (Zingmek and Rappe, 1977). Bitumen is used mainly to pave roads and is also used for coating surfaces like irrigation canal, mask asphalt for industrial flooring, electrical insulation and battery making among other uses (IPCS, 1982).

1.3 PURITY OF PETROLEUM SOLVENTS
The major impurities in petroleum solvent are compounds such as; hydrogen sulfide, mercaptan, thiophens, olefins and other unsaturated hydrocarbons. The other category of impurities are carcinogenic hydrocarbons like benzene, poly-nuclear hydrocarbon and related hetero-cyclic hydrocarbons that contain nitrogen or sulfur in the ring (IPCS, 1982).

1.4 ENVIRONMENTAL EXPOSURE LEVEL DISTRIBUTION AND TRANSFORMATION
Erhardt and Heineman, (1975), reported that low concentrations of hydrocarbons found in mussels are probably derived from petroleum hydrocarbon present in the environments. Though specific data concerning levels of petroleum solvents in air,

water, food or other environmental media are not available. It is doubtless that industrial exposure to vapour may be sometimes high due to low boiling ranges of these solvents. A lot of consumer products contain petroleum solvents; indirect exposure of general population after use is observed to certain level.

Report on distribution, transformation degradation, interaction with physical, chemical, biological factors and bio-concentration are not available, due to its complicity. Haines and Alexander,(1974) reported microbial degradation of individual petroleum hydrocarbon. Floodgate, (1972) reported the behaviour and degradation of crude oil in water.

1.5 METABOLISM

Diffusion rate, solubility in fat and the concentration gradient in individual compartment of the body determine the metabolism of petroleum solvents.

1.5.1   ABSORPTION

ACGIH, (1997), reported that cyclo-hexane is well absorbed in animals and humans through the lungs and exhaled in breath of all species studied. Gerarde, (1963), studies on rats showed that the highly volatile; C-5, C-6 and C-7 paraffins, cyclo-paraffin and aromatic hydrocarbons readily diffuse across the alveolar membrane into blood stream and are transported within minutes to the central nervous system. While longer chain homologue can pass through the alveolar membrane to a limited extent but only exert local effects. Absorption of kerosene through the skin was documented by Ritchie and colleagues, (2003).

Astrand et al, (1975) measured the alveolar air and blood concentration of white spirits in man and discovered that aromatic hydrocarbons are absorbed to a greater extent into the blood Stream than aliphatic hydrocarbon (62% and 50% respectively). Uptake values in man of benzene, and toluene and xylene had been studied by Rihimak et al., (1979) and discover that they are more readily absorbed than N-hexane. N-hexane had much lower pulmonary absorption and are excreted rapidly (Nomiyama and Nomiyana 1974).

The work of Scheuphein and Blank in 1971, showed the maximum paraffin chain length that can be absorbed through the skin is 14-Carbon atoms while aromatic hydrocarbon with greater number can still pass due to their compact structure. Absorption of vapour through the skin is very low, exposure of the whole body skin to 2250mg/m (600 ppm) of toluene was equivalent to inhalation exposure of less than 37.5 mg/m^3 (10ppm). The pattern of absorption in intestinal tract is similar to that of alveoli (IPCS, 1982).

1.5.2   DISTRIBUTION IN THE BODY

According to Bohlen et al., (1973), the tissue distribution level of inhaled anaesthetic concentration of hexane in rats depends on time of exposure and proportional to lipid content of the organ until saturation occurred. The saturation level in liver varied as its lipid level changed rapidly, hexane equally bound to some blood components.

The blood concentrations of petroleum solvents in women working at conveyor belts gluing parts of rubber footwear ranged from 2.35 ± 0.4 to 4.6 ± 0.6mg/litre at concentration in the air of 100-300mg/m^3. The blood concentration increased with numbers of years of working. (IPCS, 1982). Lipovski *et al.*, (1977) exposed rats to the solvents used in the factory at concentration in air of 300-1000mg/m^3 for 30-45 days 4h/day and found out that concentration in blood amounted to 0.45 ± 0.005 -1.2 ± 0.01mg/ litre. Pregnant wistar rats were exposed to petroleum solvents used in rubber industry at mean air concentration of 3000 ± 10mg/m^3 for 48days and 4 hours/day. The solvent was found in the blood, brain, liver, placenta, uterus and fetal tissues (Lipovski *et al.*, 1979).

Distribution of petroleum solvents was studied in 85 pregnant women working in the rubber industry, with mean air concentration of 300 ± 10mg/m^3. The average level in the blood of 46 pregnant women on whom abortion was performed was 1.27 ± 0.3mg/litre and 3.29 ± 0.6mg/kg in the embryo tissue, 39 women who gave birth to children had blood concentration of 2.5 ± 0.3mg/litre while the blood in the umbilical cord was 3.5 ± 0.3 mg/litre, the blood concentration of the new born was twice that of the mother (IPCS, 1982).

1.5.3   BIO-TRANSFORMATION

Aliphatic hydrocarbon had been shown to be bio-chemically inert in both man and rats (Williams, 1959). However few studies revealed part oxidation in mammalian tissue, Ichihara *et al*, (1969) revealed the oxidation of decane in rats and mice and conversion of hexane to hexane 2,5 dione and hexan- 2,5 –diol via methyl-n butylketone was reported by Spencer *et al*, (1978). A study in volunteers after 8hours of inhalation exposure to cyclo-hexane at concentration of 100mg/m^3 showed that 1,2 and 1,4 cyclo-hexandiol were the major metabolites,(Mraz *et al.*, 1998)

1.5.4   ELIMINATION

The elimination of the lower- boiling solvents (SBP type) is usually rapid and via the respiratory tract in both rats and humans, but ingestion of heavier solvents would include mainly elimination through feaces (Browning, 1965).

1.6.   EFFECTS ON EXPERIMENTAL ANIMALS

1.6.1   SHORT-TERM EXPOSURE

Cyclo-hexane was a weak promoter of skin tumors initiated by carcinogenic polycyclic aromatic hydrocarbon(PAH) in a mouse skin bioassay,(Gupta and Methnotra, 1990). Hine and Zuidema, (1970) reported the effects of acute toxicity of 10 samples of petroleum solvents that contained components representative of the range of hydrocarbons found in commercial petroleum solvents, four were aromatic solvents containing at least 98% aromatic hydrocarbon and 6 were aliphatic hydrocarbon containing less than 1% aromatic hydrocarbon. Acute oral inhalation and per-cutaneous toxicity; skin and eye irritancy were examined for all samples. They reported that all the solvent tested could be considered of low hazard to health except when aspirated or inhaled at high concentration. Hine and Zuidema (1970) showed that aromatic solvents were more toxic than non-aromatic having lower LD50 than aliphatic hydrocarbons.

The skin and eye irritation were also greater with aromatic hydrocarbons. The toxicity of aliphatic hydrocarbon decreases with increase in chain length. Epidermal hypertrophy, hyperplasia, hyperkeratosis and depilation were found in guinea pigs following topical application (Hoekstra and Phillips, 1963). Maximum derma-toxic effect was seen with hydrocarbon containing 14-19 carbon atoms and transition to non-dermatoxicity was seen around C21-C23 in n-paraffin. These substances had been found to have narcotic effect and cause central nervous system depression; full anaesthesia can be produced with gasoline at a concentration that is a little lower than those that cause convulsion and death (Browning, 1965). Fatal pulmonary edema and haemorrhage had been reported as a result of aspiration into lungs, the ratio of oral and intratracheal LD_{50} for kerosene was found to be 140:1 the latter being 0.2ml/kg in rats (Gerarde, 1959).

1.6.2 LONG -TERM EXPOSURE

Exposure of guinea pigs for 4hours/day, 6 days/week for a total of 65 exposures to a gasoline type solvent (boiling range 143-183^{0}C) at a concentration of 6750mg/m3, the animals were found to be restless at earlier stage followed slightly by narcotic effects, diarrhoea and albuminuria developed temporarily (Smyth and Smyth, 1928). Lipovskij, (1978) exposed matured females wistar rats to petroleum solvents vapour at a concentration of $300 \pm 8.2mg/m^2$ for 30-45 days, for 4 hours/day and found that the serotonin content of myometrium in exposed rats equaled $75.7 \pm 2.6mg/kg$ and 68.49 ± 2.5 in the control group, uterine contraction were higher and stronger in the exposed group, the uterine level of the solvent was $32.8 \pm 0.6mg/kg$ and $2.0 \pm 0.4mg/litre$ in the blood.

Miyagaki (1967) exposed five groups of 10 male mice to vapour concentrations of technical hexane of 360, 900, 1,800, 3,600 and 7,200 mg/m^3, 6th group was control, the exposure hosted 24h/day, 6 days/week for one year and observed neurogenic muscular atrophy in group with highest dosage. Neutoxicity was reported in rats exposed to high concentration of various alkyl aromatic hydrocarbon (Funmas and Hine, 1958). In a two generation inhalation reproductive study in rats exposed throughout the study to 0, 500, 2000 or 700ppm cyclo-hexane. No compound related adverse effect was observed at 500ppm. At 2000ppm the only adverse effect was diminished or no alerting response. At 7000ppm reduction in mean body weight for P1 and F1 females and F1 males as well as reduced mean pulp weight for F1 and F2 litters were observed, (Kreckmann et al., 1998a). Assumed pregnant rabbits were exposed to 0, 500, 20000, 7000 ppm cyclo-hexane on day 6 to 8 of gestation. The animals were sacrificed at day 29. No maternal or developmental toxicity was observed in this study, (Kreckmann et al.,1998b).

1.6.3 EFFECTS ON AQUATIC ANIMALS

Khan et al, (1995) studied on contaminating effects of petroleum hydrocarbon on fish species showed that minnows and mullets were found to accumulate aromatic hydrocarbon to much as 3-4mg/gm wet weight of the fish, the mullet absorbed the hydrocarbon slowly and degrade them more readily, but the minnows absorbed them more rapidly and retained the compounds. For as much as two weeks after being transferred to uncontaminated water from sea water. Dede and Kaglo, (2001) reported that some fishes can store aromatic hydrocarbon and pass them to higher trophic level. Kennicutt and Sweet, (1992), discovered spoil related contamination in the intertidal limpet Maaela concinna, two years after release of 600,000 litres of diesel fuel into Arthur Harbour in the Antarctic peninsula.

The fish, *Fundulus heteroclittus* collected from the Wild Harbour marsh, where diesel fuel spill occurred in 1969 was found to contain up 75ppm of petroleum hydrocarbon in its tissue several years later (Sabo and Stageman, 1977). Subtle changes have been reported in fish that are both chronically or briefly exposed. The toxic effect depend on amount of oil spilled the area covered by the oil and the chemical composition of the oil, the fish species and the duration of the oil on the fish (Kihnhold, 1980). The exposure of tilapia (*Oreochromis niloticus*) fingerlings to water soluble fraction of Nigeria diesel fuel showed mortality at low concentration. Histo-pathological study of the gills showed structural abnormality as elongation, fusion and hyper-plasia of the lamellae (Dede and Kaglo, 2001). The toxicity of the water soluble fraction of diesel fuel to tilapia fingerling was supported by the study of Kihnhold, (1980).

The pH of the water was within the Federal Environmental Protection Agency range for sustenance of aquatic life, contribution of pH to toxicity is uncertain. The dissolved content of oxygen in the water soluble fraction was below the acceptable level for water quality sustenance. The low oxygen tension has been shown to be due to diversion of oxygen to the oxidation of the organic pollutant. Oxygen stress and consequently respiratory stress which was beyond what the fish can withstand became obvious. Water soluble fraction of crude oil was shown to impart the same oxygen stress. The elongation and hyper-plasia of the gill might be induced by oxygen stress (Dede and kaglo, 2001). Similar reports have been documented in shrimps and catfish (Baden, 1982).

1.7   EFFECTS ON MAN
1.7.1 CONTROLLED EXPOSURES
Skin irritation and defecting was reported by Ritchie *et al*, (2003), after patch testing petroleum solvents with various boiling ranges on the skin of human volunteers; the impact was found to correlate with the boiling ranges which decrease with increase in boiling range. The range that includes kerosene was found to be of primary irritants and the higher the aromatic content the greater the irritation, higher tolerance was found in the skin of the Negroes than Caucasians. Pre-existing skin disease favours the increase susceptibility of skin to these effects. Ritchie *et al*, (2003), reported the result of dermatological study of ball-bearing workers (n=79) who were daily exposed to kerosene as asymptomatic 16%; erythematic 65%, eczematous 15% and defecting dermatitis 4%. Undiluted refined kerosene was applied in an occluded patch-test, burning sensation was developed after one hour, after 2 hours slight erythema and the skin was tender and red after 7 hours, after 12

hours, the burning sensation subsided but a large tense bulla red appeared surrounded by small scattered vesicles. This changed to a large flaccid purulent bulla later which broke early (Fagani and Ogino, 1973).

David *et al.*, (1960) reported the exposure of human volunteers for 30 minutes to concentration of petrol of 900, 2250 or 4,500 mg/m^3 in air, itching and burning of the eyes were apparent at highest concentration while fewer symptoms were noted at lower concentrations. Vapour of hydrocarbons can be detected at low concentrations but unpleasant odour and irritation became apparent at high concentration, human sensory data were often limiting factors in establishing exposure limit (Carpenter *et al*, 1977). Chronic exposure had been found to be probably associated with tightness of chest and breathing difficulties (Ritchie *et al.*, 2003).

1.7.2 EPIDEMIOLOGICAL STUDIES
1.7.2.0 OCCUPATIONAL EXPOSURES

Okoro *et al.*, (2006), investigated haemato-toxic implications of exposure to petroleum fumes through inhalation in fuel attendants in Calabar metropolis in Nigeria, a total of about 400 subjects (200 males and 200 females) between 18-30 years. The subjects were divided into two groups; those that have been exposed up to 2 years (T1) and those that have been exposed for more than 2 years (T2). They reported that the odds of a subject becoming anaemic increases progressively from control to T1 and it was highest at T2. Female subjects were more likely to become anaemic than male counterparts in the exposed groups, they concluded that petroleum fumes causes depression of total white blood cells count as well as red blood cell count in correlation to the duration of exposure.

The toxic components especially those in petroleum fumes have been reported to change blood chemistry and induce anaemia by causing bone marrow hypoplasia, benzene had been known to cause haematological changes ranging from pancytopenia to total bone marrow aplasia and xylene is also reported to cause leukocytopaenia (d'Azevedo *et al*, 1996). Metals like lead and volatile nitrates had been shown to have harmful effect on the bone marrow (Okoro *et al*, 2006).

1.7.2.1 NEURO-PATHOLOGICAL EFFECTS

Carney, (2005), reported that aromatic hydrocarbons in petrol and other inhalants affects the fronto-cortical areas and low basal ganglia networks on the brain, thus leads to euphoria, relaxation, double vision and slurred speech and hallucination. Heavy exposure to leaded petrol can affect the cerebellum. Exposure of car painters over many years to low concentration of solvents containing mixtures of toluene, xylene, butyl acetate and white spirit was found to be associated with an increased incidence of sleep disturbance, absentmindedness, falling sleep while watching television and headaches. Lower peripheral nerve conduction velocities, psychomotor impairment and personality changes were more common in exposed than in control subjects (Seppalaiman *et al*, 1978). The average period of exposure was 17 years and the estimated exposure was 300mg/m^3. Significant difference was found between exposed and unexposed groups in the incidence and prevalence of psychiatric symptoms, psychological test results, especially attention and sensorimotor speed, and on electroencephalograms.

Franco *et al* (1979) reported sensory and peripheral motor conduction disturbances where exposure to cyclo-hexane had occurred, n-hexane and n-heptane were also found to cause poly-neuropathy, complaint of insomnia, irritability and other non-specific CNS symptoms. A study of 18 workers exposed to glue containing 75.6% cyclo-hexane, 12% toluene and 0.9% hexane, showed that concentration of airbore cyclo-hexane ranging from 5-211ppm did not have any adverse effect on the peripheral nervous system, (Yuasa *et al.*, 1996).

1.7.2.2 EFFECT ON REPRODUCTIVE FUNCTIONS

Koschier, (1999), reported that kerosene dose not have a measurable effect on human reproduction or development. Gynecological studies were conducted on more than 5,000 female operators in rubber plants (petroleum solvents vapour in the air between 250-350mg/m3) by Beskrovmaja *et al*, (1979). High frequency of metrorrhagia and disturbance in menstrual cycle were observed in worker with more than 5 years experience. As the period of service increased, a reduction in the frequency of miscarriages was observed, which was interpreted by the author or possible adaptation. Disturbances of ovarian functions were noted in 2.4% of the workers examined.

Examination of vaginal smears of 184 female gluers in the rubber industry (18-38 years old) revealed a disturbance of the ovarian function with reduced oestrogen secretion in 21.7% (10.49% in control group). After ten years of service the percentage doubled after five years observation. It was found that sensitivity of ovaries to gonadotrophins were reduced as there were significant changes in secretion of FSH (Follicular Stimulating Hormones) and LH (Leutenizing Hormones) (Noviko *et al*, 1979). Hypolactin was observed in women working in rubber industry who were exposed to petroleum solvents vapour concentration of $300mg/m^3$, the severity is related to number of years in service, and hydrocarbons were found in milk of women examined and serotonin content in the blood were lower than the control, it was assumed that this was effect of petroleum solvents on lactation mechanism via the hypothalamus and the serotonergic system (Noviko *et al*, 1979).

1.7.2.3 EFFECT ON THE SKIN

Sumamur and Susiantiwemas, (1979), reported that the study of 54 gasoline and diesel station workers; only dryness, chapping and reddening of the skin were found. The most common health effect associated with chronic and repeated kerosene exposure is dermatitis,(Ritchie *et al.*, 2003).

1.7.3 CLINICAL STUDIES
1.7.3.1 DERMAL EXPOSURE

Jee *et al.*, (1986), reported the result of a dermatological study of ball-bearing workers (n=79) exposed on a daily basis to kerosene as follows; asymptomatic 16%, erythematic 65%, eczematous 15% and defecting dermatitis 4%. The defecting action

16

on the skin and repeating exposure cause injury to the horny layer; this makes the skin more susceptible to other irritants, sensitizing agents and bacteria, it also cause progressive dermatitis which could lead to eczema as seen in workers in garages or automobile repair shop who wash their hands with petrol or kerosene (Tagami and Ogino, 1973), these effects on skin decrease with higher boiling range.

Cases in which gasoline or kerosene randomly contact with skin for prolonged period occur mainly in children or in unconscious accident, victims. When clothing has become soaked with the solvent. Lesion start with burning sensation, formation of small and large blister, to extensive epidermolysis which became muco-purulent in a few days (Browning, 1965). Hayhurst, (1936), reported that gasoline may be absorbed through the skin in toxic quantities if large areas of skin were exposed in case of extensive epidermolysis.

1.7.3.2 EFFECTS OF INHALATION

Browning, (1965) showed that the effect of acute massive over exposure to gasoline vapour is mainly narcosis with loss of consciousness and possibly convulsion which may be fatal, octane is known to cause rapid and deep narcosis while pentane and hexane have less narcotic effect, but exert a paralytic effect on the central nervous system and respiratory system along with heptane. In gradual overexposure, the symptom is preceeded with eye irritation, irritation of the respiratory tract, dizziness, headache and sense of drunkenness.

According to Wang, (1961), the margin of safety between narcosis and respiratory arrests is very narrow in exposure to high concentration of gasoline. Acute occupational poisoning by gasoline vapour is mostly caused by entering unpurged Gasoline tanks, exposure to high concentrations may also occur in car accidents when victim are trapped or unconscious. Histo-pathological changes found in the subjects who died after exposure to high concentration of gasoline vapour include: necrosis of alveolar wall, haemorrhages or effusion in internal organs and serous cavities, liver and kidney showed bad degeneration, hyperemia and oedema of the brain and myelin sheat swelling (Browning, 1965; Machle, 1941). Non specific symptom of the nervous system and digestive tract are evident in long term exposure to low concentration, the reproductive organ may be affected in woman (Schtman *et al*, 1999).

1.7.3.3 EFFECTS OF INGESTION

Accidental ingestion of petroleum distillates in the ranges of petroleum solvents is an important cause of poisoning in children, in most cases it is caused by gasoline and kerosene. Coughing, choking and gagging are often noted at the time of ingestion. Respiratory embarrassment may be present early indicating aspiration which occur in 95% of children, epigastric discomfort which lead to vomiting and another risk of aspiration (Gerarde, 1963). Aspiration of 1-2ml of kerosene may cause fatal pulmonary changes, but if aspiration does not occur much larger quantities could be tolerated, children are more susceptible than adults (Browning, 1969; Hansen, 1959).

1.7.3.4 GENE TOXICITY

An ncrease in cytogenic changes (chromosomal aberrations in peripheral lymphocytes and bone marrow micronuclei) has been reported in a limited study of workers exposed to a mixture of kerosene, bunker fuels white spirit and xylene, (Hogstedt *et al.*, 1981). However the mixed exposure precludes any specific conclusions and the results did not correlate with the effects of kerosene only.

1.7.3.5 CARCINOGENICITY

An excess of lung cancer was seen in a large cohort of Japanese workers exposed to kerosene, diesel oil, crude petroleum and mineral oil, (IARC, 1989). In another Japanese study, an excess of stomach cancer was observed amongst workers who were exposed to kerosene, machine oil or grease,(IARC, 1989). Three case-control studies found an association between lung cancer and the use of kerosene stoves for cooking amongst women in Honkong; however , no distinction was made between exposure to kerosene per se and exposure to its combustion products, (IARC,1989).

1.8   EFFECTS OF PETROLEUM ADDITIVES
1.8.1 EFFECTS OF LEAD (TETRAETHYL LEAD)

Studies on both animals and humans indicate that lipids metabolism is altered in chronic lead exposure, though the pathophysiological mechanism involved are not completely understood. Lead has been shown to accelerate lipid oxidation in the presence of haemoglobin or Fe^{2+} (Adonaylo, 1999; Quinlan *et al.*, 1988). Lead was also shown to enhance Fe^{2+} initiated lipid oxidation in liposomes, erythrocytes, microsomal fractions and rat brain homogenates. Altered fatty acid composition of erythrocytes membranes has also been demonstrated in chronic lead exposure (Quinlan *et al*, 1988).

Few published reports exist about lead poisoning in developing countries like Nigeria. Ademuyiwa *et al*, (2005), investigated the distribution of blood lipids in 110 male subjects in Abeokuta, Nigeria, who have been shown to be occupationally exposed to lead. The artisans include auto-mechanic, petrol station attendants, drivers, spare part dealers, majority of the artisans spent an average of 11 hours per day in their workshop. They found out that total cholesterol was between 1.5 and 2.0 times higher in artisans than control, and LDL- cholesterol was between 1.6 and 2.4 times higher than control while HDL-cholesterol and triglycerides were not affected. They observed a significant positive correlation between blood lead and total cholesterol level and blood lead LDL-cholesterol and concluded that lead exposure increases blood cholesterol

OTHER EFFECTS OF LEAD

EPA (2005), reports showed that lead has adverse effects on organs. Lead causes damage to the kidney, liver, brain, nerves and other organs. Exposure to lead may also cause osteoporosis and reproductive disorder. Excessive exposure to lead causes seizures, mental retardation, behavioural disorders, memory problems and mood changes. It also causes learning defect in children and lower their intelligent quotient (EPA, 2005). Lead causes high blood pressure and increases heart diseases in many men, may also cause anaemia (EPA, 2005).

1.8.2 EFFECTS OF 2,2,4 TRIMETHYLPENTANE

2,2,4 Trimethylpentane is released to the environment through the manufacture, use and disposal of products associated with the petroleum and gasoline industry. During an accident, 2,2,4 – trimethylpentane penetrated the skin of human which caused necrosis of the skin and tissue in the hand and required surgery (USDHHS, 1993). No other information is available on the acute (short term) effects in humans. Irritation of the lungs, edema, and hemorrhage have been reported in rodents acutely exposed by inhalation and injection (Clayton and Clayton, 1981).

No information is available on the chronic (long term) exposure on reproductive, developmental, or carcinogenic effects of 2,2,4trimethylpentane in humans while rats exposed chronically via gavage and inhalation has shown kidney and liver effects (USDHHS, 1993).

1.8.3 EFFECTS OF CUMENE

Cumene is used in variety of petroleum products as thinner for example, lacquers and enamel. It is used as component of high octane fuels and it is used in the manufacture of phenols, octane, acetophenone and methylstyrene (USDHHS, 1993; Sitting, 1985). Cumene is a constituent of crude oils and finished fuels. It is released to the environment as a result of its production and processing from petroleum refining, evaporation and combustion of petroleum products. The most probable route of human exposure is through inhalation of contaminated oil and consumption of contaminated food or water (USDHHS, 1993).

No information is available on chronic exposure in humans. Inhalation studies have been reported to increase liver, kidney and adrenal weights in rats, Increased kidney weight was observed in rats chronically exposed to cumene via gavages (USEPA, 1999). No information is available on the reproductive or developmental effects of cumene in humans, inhalation studies in rat and rabbits showed no significant adverse effect on reproduction or fetal development (USEPA, 1999). No effects on sperm were observed in male rats exposed by inhalation (USEPA, 1997). No report on the carcinogenic effect of cumene (USEPA, 1997).

1.9. EFFECTS OF PETROLEUM PRODUCTS ON PLASMA LIPIDS

Only few works has been done on effects of petroleum products on lipid metabolism. Achuba, (2005), reported that ingestion of crude petroleum contaminated diet impose a reciprocal relationship between HDL-cholesterol and LDL -cholesterol in the plasma of rabbit. Ingestion of petroleum has been shown to cause reduction in blood glucose. This may shift the demand for metabolic substrate to lipid (Ben-David et al., 2001), this may explain the significant decrease in the blood level of triglycerides in rabbit fed with petroleum contaminated diet relative to control (Achuba, 2005).

Achuba and Osakwe, (2003), reported that ingestion of petroleum hydrocarbon induce oxidative stress through generation of free radical. Free radical generation with subsequent oxidative modification that leads to lipid per-oxidation that damage macro-molecules such as DNA, and proteins, (Souza et al, 1999).

1.10 EFFECTS OF DYSLIPIDEMIA

Dyslipidemia is a strong predictor of cardiovascular diseases and it has been shown to be co-risk factor in hypertension along with obesity and diabetes (Ruben et al., 2006). Renal insufficiency has been associated with abnormalities in lipoprotein metabolism in both early and late stages of chronic renal failure (Crook et al, 2003). In animal models alterations in lipids metabolism and action led to macrophages activation and infiltration in the kidney with resultant tubulo-interstitial and endothelial cell injury (Crook et al, 2003). Calorioso et al, (1999) conducted a trial of pravastatin in 30 hypertensive hyper-cholesterolemia subjects and demonstrated that compared with placebo treatment, pravastin insgnificantly decrease systolic, diastolic and pulse pressures, and blunted the blood pressure increase induced by the cold pressor test.

Atherogenic lipid abnormalities cause endothelia dysfunction, a dysfunctional endothelium will express impaired nitric oxide production and activity, as well as alteration in endothelin - 1 and endothelin A and B-receptor expression (Ruben et al, 2006). Lipid abnormalities and insulin resistance have been associated with sympathetic hypertension which may play a role in development of hypertension (Egan, 2003). Shen et al, (2003) reported that hypertension may be late stage manifestation, arising secondary to derangement of other components of the metabolic syndrome, such as dsylipidemia, while Ruben et al., (2006), concluded from their prospective study that there is an independent relationship between increased plasma lipid level and incident of hypertension and that hypertension may represent early manifestation of the atherosclerosis process.

1.10.1 MECHANISM THROUGH WHICH DYSLIPIDEMIA ACTS AS CARDIOVASCULAR DISEASES RISK FACTOR.

Mechanisms by which dyslipidemia exert its effect as cardiovascular disease risk factor is not yet well established, but there are two mechanisms based on past studies. In the first mechanism, this is based on oxidative modification that occur to LDL-cholesterol particles in the plasma and the effect of these modification on the routes of elimination of these particles (Steinberg and Witzum, 1990). The oxidative modification of the LDL-cholesterol causes macrophages to take up LDL particles through a receptor – independent pathway and in this way increasing the atherogenicity of LDL particles. These modification also affect HDL particles (Austin et al, 1990).

The second mechanism is much less established. It is based on the theory that procoagulant enzymatic complex assembly and activity (e.g prothrombinase) require a surface and there is some evidence that lipoprotein particles provide this surface, according to Bradley *et al*, 1989). Also that apoliprotein A, a fraction of LDL may interfere with proper fibrinolysis (Mile *et al*, 1989).

Alteration in platelets function with elevated plasma lipid level have been documented in either animal model as in hypercholesteronic rabbit or human. Nofer *et al* (1997) reported that LDL increases cardiovascular disease risk by altering platelet metabolism resulting in increase platelet responsiveness to activating agents, which leads to a significant drop in intra-platelet pH and inhibition of the agonist induced Na^+/H^+ exchange. Though this theory needs further study.

CHAPTER TWO

2.0 RESEARCH METHODOLOGY

This study was designed for the in-vivo measurement of blood pressure and heart rate and to assess the effects on plasma lipids profile after administration of some petroleum solvents and their water soluble fractions (WSF). 35 experimental rats with average weight of 150grams before administration were anaesthetized, dissected and canulated for blood pressure and heart rate recording, blood was collected for plasma lipids profile analysis after three weeks of oral administration of petroleum products; diesel, kerosene, petrol and their water soluble fractions (WSF) .

2.1 MATERIALS AND METHODS
2.1.2.ANIMALS AND FEEDING PROTOCOL

Experimental rats; male Wistar Rats*(Rattus norvegicus)* of about 14 weeks old were bought from Anatomy Department of University of Ibadan were used for this study. They were acclimatized for a period of four weeks, and for the duration of the experiment in a well ventilated cages in the Laboratory Animal Centre of the College of Medicine, University of Lagos. The animals had average weight of 150 grammes, before the commencement of administration.

The animals were fed with mouse cube bought from Lives Stocks Feeds Plc. Ikeja, Lagos. The composition of the feed was as follows:

Protein   -   21.0%
Fiber   -   5.0%
Fat   -   5.0%
Av. Phosphorous   -   0.6%
Energy   -   2640 kcal/kg

The animals had free access to food and water throughout the study.

2.1.2 SOURCE OF THE PETROLEUM PRODUCTS AND THEIR WATER SOLUBLE FRACTIONS.

Petroleum products; diesel, kerosene and petrol were bought from Total Filling Station at Mushin, Lagos.

To extract the water soluble fractions, equal volumes (100 ml) of water and each solvents were measured into a bottle at a time and covered then shaken thoroughly until the mixture had uniform appearance and then poured into a separating funnel and allowed to stand for 24 hours to allow clear separation of liquid-water interface, then the water portion was carefully collected. This was done for each petroleum product. The concentration of dissolved portion was determined as follows:

Water soluble fraction of diesel   -   0.25% v/v
Water soluble fraction of kerosene -   0.28% v/v
Water soluble fraction of petrol   -   0.50% v/v

2.1.3 ADMINISTRATION (ROUTE AND DURATION)

The petroleum solvents and their water soluble fractions were administered orally for a period of three weeks (21 days).

Group I   - Control was given placebo (normal water).
Group IIa - was given 4 ml/kg of pure diesel.
Group IIb - was given 14 ml/kg of water soluble fraction(WSF) of diesel.
Group IIIa - was given 4 ml/kg of pure kerosene.
Group IIIb - was given 14 ml/Kg of water soluble fraction(WSF) of kerosene.
Group Iva - was given 4 ml/kg of pure petrol.
Group IVb - was given 7 ml/kg of water soluble fraction of petrol.

The oral administration of these solvents was achieved by withdrawing the desired volume into syringe fitted with bulb tipped gastric gavage needle, the animal was then held by the skin behind its neck which caused the mouth to open. The cannula was passed from the mouth onto the stomach through the oesophagus carefully to avoid aspiration. This was done for 21 days.

2.1.4 APPARATUS

i.   Grass 7D polygraph (Grass Instruments Limited, Quincy, Massachussets) and pressure transducer (P23LD Statham Hato Rey Inc.) They are used in the recording of arterial blood pressure and heart rate .

ii.   Tracheal cannula; used to ensure proper ventilation.

iii.   Arterial cannula with 2-way tap and lock used for cannulating femoral artery and serve as connecting medium to transducer for determining blood pressure and heart rate.

iv.   Syringe and needles; 1ml, 2ml, & 5ml for administration of anaesthetic agents, filling the transducer with and blood samples collection.

v.   Oral Cannula: For administration of petroleum solvents.

vi.   Rat Weighing Balance (Divet by Salter), for checking the weight of the rats.

vii.   Flasks and beakers.

viii. Dissecting boards and pins and dissecting kits used for spreading and holding the animal in place for dissection and dissecting the anaesthetized animals.

ix.   Bull Dog Clips: used for occluding the femoral artery during cannulation.

x.   Centrifuge machine, centrifuge tubes and capillary tubes for centrifuging the blood so that the plasma could be collected for lipid analysis and to determine the packed cell volume,

xi.   Water Bath. For warming the anaesthetic agent.

xii.   Sartorus balance. Used in weighing out the constituents of the anaesthetic agent.

xiii. Cotton wool for soaking up the blood from point of dissection.

Xiv   Animal weighing balance; for weighing the animals.

2.1.5 REAGENTS

Heparinised normal saline containing 0.9% sodium chloride and 1% heparin was used to keep exposed areas moist during dissection and fill the transducer.

Urethane/Alpha chloralose – 20% w/v (BDH, Chemical, Poole, England). This mixture was weighed out on the satoris balance and a solution was made using distilled water in a flask. It was used as anaesthesia.

Distilled water was used to dissolve various chemicals.

Heparin for preparing heparinized normal saline.

2.2 METHODOLOGY

The experiment was carried out as follows:

Oral administration of petroleum solvents and their water soluble fractions.

Anaesthetizing, dissection and cannulation of the animals.

Recording of the blood pressure and heart rate.

Blood chemistry analysis.

2.2.1 PREPARATION OF THE ANIMALS FOR EXPERIMENT

The animals were anaesthesized with a mixture of urethane 20% (w/v) and alpha chloralose 1% in distilled water. The urethane was prepared to 20% instead of usual 25% to avoid hypotension in the animals, because urethane could induce hypotension on cardiovascular system. The anaesthesia was administered at a dose of 5ml/kg intraperitoneally and when necessary additional 0.5 ml was given to maintain surgical anaesthesia.

After the administration of the anaesthetic agent, the animal was left for some minutes until its effects sets in. the degree of anaesthesia was assessed as a lack of response towards painful stimuli, diminished muscular tone, absence of corneal reflex and presence of normal breathing in term of frequency and amplitude.

2.2.2 DISSECTION AND CANNULATION

The anaesthetized animal was placed on dissecting board with the ventral surface facing upwards and its limbs pinned down. A fold of skin was cut off with a pair of scissors from the upper part of the sternum and extended towards the base of the jaw in order to expose the underlying connective tissue. The trachea was exposed by blunt dissection and loop of ligature was placed on it. The exposed trachea was semi-transected between two tracheal rings half way in the neck. A polythene cannula with an internal diameter similar to the trachea was inserted and firmly tied in place with the ligature. The cannulation was done to avoid blockade and aspiration of fluids into the lungs.

A fold of skin was held up at the lower limb using forceps and a sharp pair of scissors were used to make a blunt skin incision to expose the underlying connective tissue. The adipose tissue and fascia were separated carefully to expose the femoral vessels, the femoral artery was carefully separated. The distal end of the femoral artery was tied while the proximal end was occluded with bull dog clip. Incision was made close to the distal end and cannulated by using polythene cannula attached to 5 ml syringe filled with heparinized normal saline solution. The bull dog clip was carefully removed while the catheter was further pushed into the vessel. The distal part of the cannula was then tied to hold the catheter in place. Blood was dpuren through the cannula and flushed back with heparinized normal saline to ensure that the cannula was not blocked(Anigbogu and Adigun, 1987).

2.2.3 BALANCING THE POLYGRAPH
The polygraph (Grass Instrument Ltd, Quincy, Massachusetts, USA) was switched on and all channels were put on standby for 5 minutes after which the channel to be used of the Grass 7D Polygraph was switched to 'on'. The D/C driver amplifier of the Grass 7D polygraph was set on calibration and the baseline knob was used to position the recording pen on the recording paper, this was the recording baseline. The pen recorder was adjusted to standard deflection of 2cm/100mv.

The control knob was then set on 'use' pre amplifier was set at 1mv/cm. After this the polygraph was ready for use and all the while, the pressure transducer has been connected to the polygraph.

2.2.4 BLOOD PRESSURE MEASUREMENT
The calibration of the pressure transducer was done using a manometer. The manometer pressure was raised on a step-wise manner of 20 mmHg and deflection was mark on recording paper. This calibration record was used to calculate the systolic and diastolic blood pressure of rats. The arterial cannula was cannulated to the Stathon P.23 ID strain gauge pressure transducer. The transducer convert mechanical energy into electrical energy, which is in turn amplified and converted back to mechanical energy indicated by pen deflection.

The peak of the pen deflection was taken as the systolic blood pressure while the lower point was taken as diastolic blood pressure. The mean arterial pressure(MAP) was obtained from the reading using the formular; MAP= Diastolic pressure + 1/3 Pulse pressure(DP + 1/3PP)mmHg, (Anigbogu and Adigun 1996).

2.2.5DETERMINATION OF PACKED CELL VOLUME
This was determined using the microhaematocrit method. It was described by cheesbrough (2002).

The rat's blood to be determined is drawn up into the heparinized capillary tubes until about three-quarter of the tube. The outside of the tube was then cleaned with cotton wool to remove blood. The ends of the capillary tubes were closed with plasticine. These tubes were then fixed into the microhaematocrit centrifuge and spinned for five minutes at a speed of 3000rpm. The haematocrit was then immediately read using a micro-haematocrit reader and the result expressed as percentages

2.2.6 PLASMA LIPIDS PROFILE ANALYSIS
The blood samples were collected into heparinized sample bottles. The blood sample was centrifuged at 5000g for ten minutes to remove the plasma.

TOTAL CHOLESTEROL
This was analyzed using BIOLABO SA CHOD-PAP reagents (Ref 80106).

Blank   -   1ml of the reagent was pippeted into the test tube.

Standard-   1ml of the reagent was pippeted and 10μL of the standard.

Sample- 1ml of the reagent was pippeted and 10μl of the sample was added.

Each test tube was thoroughly mixed and incubated for 5 minutes at 37^0C.

The absorbance of the sample and standard were measured against blank at 500nm using spectrometer (Allain *et al*, 1974).

cholesterol conc. = $\dfrac{\text{Absorbance of the sample}}{\text{Absorbance of the standard}}$ x standard conc. (mmol/L)

HDL –CHOLESTEROL

This was analysed using BIOLABO S-HDL-CHOLESTEROL (PTA) – reagents.

The sample was precipitated to form supernatant as follows using macro-method.

Formation of the supernatant: 1ml of the sample was pippeted to a centrifuge tube, then 100μl of the precipitant was added and mixed vigorously, it was allowed to stand for ten minutes at room temperature. Then it was centrifuge at 1500g for 15 minutes.The reagent and supernatants were allowed to stand at room temperature.

HDL-cholesterol Assay

Blank- 1ml of the reagents was pippeted on to test tube and 25μl of distilled water was added.

Standard – 1ml of the reagents and 25μl of the standard (100 ml/dl) were pippeted into test tube.

Assay – 1ml of the reagents was pippeted into test tube and 25μl of the supernatant was added.

Each was mixed and allowed to stand for five minutes at 37^0C. The absorbance of the assay and standard were measured against blank at 500 nm using spectrometer, (Badimon *et al*, 1990; Gotto, 1988).

HDL   = $\dfrac{\text{Abs (Assay)}}{\text{Abs (Standard)}}$ x Standard Conc. x 1.1 (mmol/L)

TRIGLYCERIDES

This was analysed using BIOLAB reagents – GPO method.

Blank- 1ml of the reagent and 10μl distilled water were pippeted into test tube.

Standard- 1ml of the reagent was pippeted and 10μl of the standard plasma was added.

Sample - 10μl of the sample was added to 1ml of the reagent in the test tube.

The test tubes were mixed and allowed to stand for 5minutes at 37^0C. The absorbance of the standard and sample were read against blank at 500nm using spectrometer.

Result = $\dfrac{\text{Abs (Assay)}}{\text{Abs (Standard)}}$ x Standard conc. (mmol/L)

(Tietz, 1995).

LDL CHOLESTEROL
LDL cholesterol from each sample was calculated using the formular.
LDL cholestrol = Total cholesterol – (TG)/2.2 + HDL-cholesterol (mmol/L)

2.2.6 STATISTICAL ANALYSIS
All results obtained were presented as tables to enable easy assessment. Comparison of control and test values to facilitate understanding of data and analysis through data summary like mean, standard deviation, standard error of mean (SEM)

$$\text{Mean } (x) = \frac{\sum x}{n}$$

$$\text{SD} = \frac{\sum (x - x)^2}{n-1}$$

$$\text{SEM} = \frac{\sqrt{SD}}{n - 1}$$

DATA ANALYSIS
The standard t-test was used to analyse the level of significant between the control group and treated groups.

The level of significance for the t-test was taken as $P < 0.05$

CHAPTER THREE
RESULTS

3.1 BLOOD PRESSURE AND HEART RATE

The mean of blood pressure parameters of each group is shown in table 3.1.

There was no observed difference in systolic blood pressure except water WSF-diesel(80 ± 10.96mmHg, p-value <0.05) that was significantly lower than contro(120 ± 4.90mmHg).

The diastolic blood pressure was lower in treated groups but only WSF-diesel(52.4 ± 9.09 mmHg) $P<0.01$, pure kerosene(86.4 ± 2.64 mmHg) $P<0.05$ and pure petrol(72 ± 6.40mmHg) p-value<0.01 were significant. While pure diesel(88 ± 2.53mmHg), WSF-kerosene(116 ± 3.85mmHg) and WSF-petrol(82 ± 6.00 mmHg) were not significantly lower, p >0.05.

The mean pulse pressure was significantly higher in pure diesel group(39 ± 2.65 mmHg) $P< 0.05$, pure kerosene group(39 ± 0.77mmHg) $P<0.01$, pure petrol group(37 ± 2.32mmhg) $P<0.05$ and WSF-petrol(37 ± 2.32 mmHg) $P < 0.05$. WSF-kerosene (29 ± 1.00 mmHg) $P>0.05$ was insignificantly higher, while the WSF-diesel, (21.2 ± 4.59 mmHg) was insignificantly lower with p-value >0.05, compared with control(25 ± 1.95 mmHg).

The mean arterial blood pressure was lower in all treated groups, but only WSF-diesel(61 ± 9.3 mmHg) $P < 0.01$ and pure petrol group(84 ± 6.87mmHg) $P<0.05$, were significant compared to control (103 ± 2.61mmHg).

The heart rate was significantly higher in all treated groups compared to control(368 ± 3.6beat/min); pure diesel(408 ± 849beats/min) $P<0.01$, pure kerosene(411 ± 6.46beat/min) $P<0.001$, WSF-kerosene(414 ± 8.05beat/min) $P<0.001$, petrol(423 ± 6.6 beat/min) $P<0.001$ and WSF-petrol(400.8 ± 7.68beats/min) $P<0.01$. While WSF-diesel (390 ± 14.4beats/min) $P>0.05$, was insignificant.

TABLE 3.1: TABLE OF VALUES SHOWING THE EFFECTS OF PURE DIESEL, KEROSENE AND PETROL AND THEIR WATER SOLUBLE FRACTIONS ON BLOOD PRESSURE AND HEART RATE

Parameters		Control	Pure Diesel	WSF Diesel	Pure Kerosene	WSF Kerosene	Pure Petrol	WSF Petrol
Systolic Blood Pressure (mmHg)	Mean	120	127	80	125.2	116	109.6	118
	SEM ±	4.90	4.8	10.96	2.92	3.85	8.13	4.10
	P.Value		NS	*	NS	NS	NS	NS
Diastolic Blood Pressure (mmHg)	Mean	95	88	52.4	86.4	87	72.4	82
	SEM ±	1.95	2.53	9.09	2.64	4.80	6.40	6.00
	P.Value		NS	**	**	NS	*	NS
Pulse Pressure (mmHg)	Mean	25	39	21.2	39	29	37	37
	SEM ±	4.07	2.65	4.59	0.77	1.00	2.32	2.32
	P.Value		*	NS	**	NS	*	*
Mean Arterial Pressure (mmHg)	Mean	103	101	61.4	99.4	96.2	84.8	94
	SEM ±	2.61	3.23	9.3	2.69	4.43	6.87	5.32
	P.Value		NS	**	NS	NS	*	NS
Heart Rate (Beat/.min)	Mean	368	408	390	411.6	414	423	400.8
	SEM ±	3.6	8.94	14.45	6.64	8.05	6.6	7.68
	P.Value		**	NS	***	***	***	**

Significant level: *P-value <0.05, **P-value <0.01, ***P-value <0.001, NS- Non-significant P-value >0.05.   SEM- Standard Error of Mean.

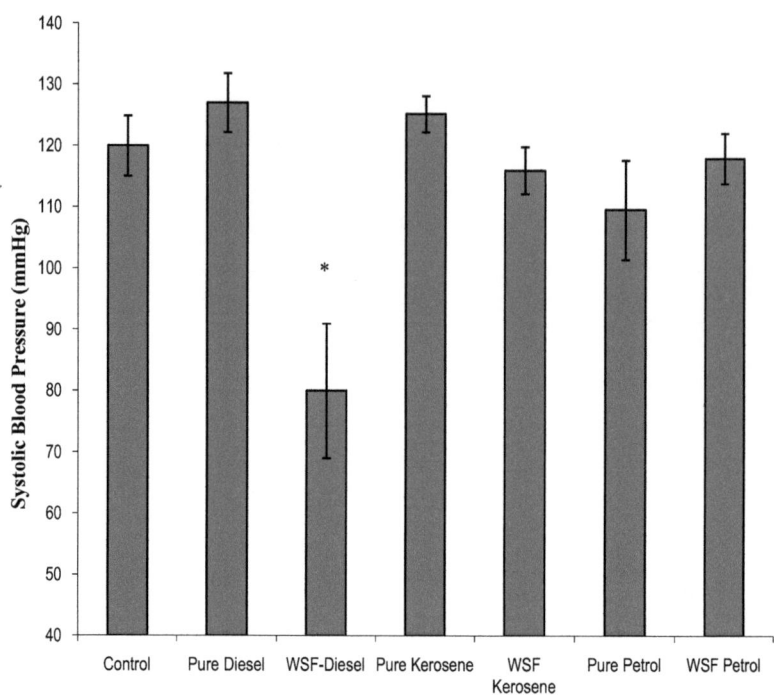

Fig.3.1.1: Bar chart Showing the effect of petroleum products and their water soluble fractions on systolic blood pressure. * = Significant ,P<0.05

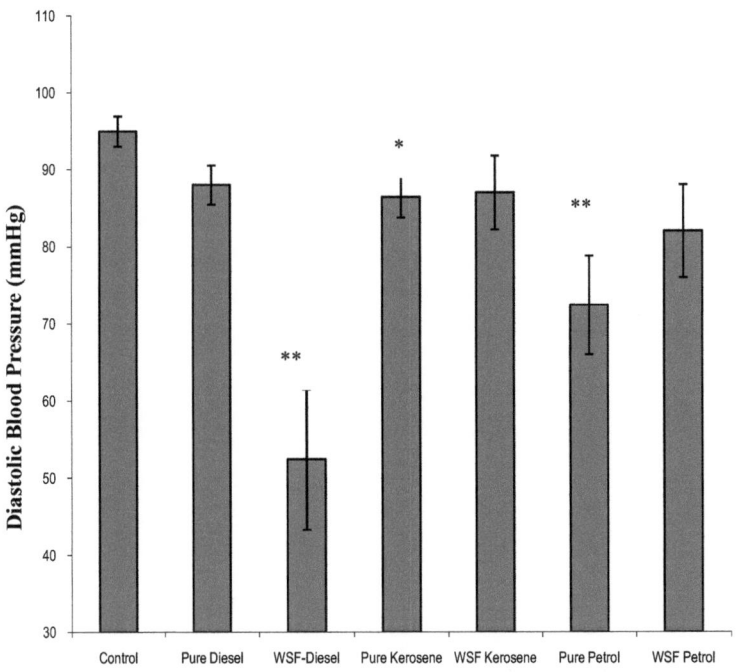

Fig.3.1.2: Bar chart Showing the effect of petroleum products and their water soluble fractions on diastolic blood pressure.
* = P <0.05, Significant. ** = P < 0.01

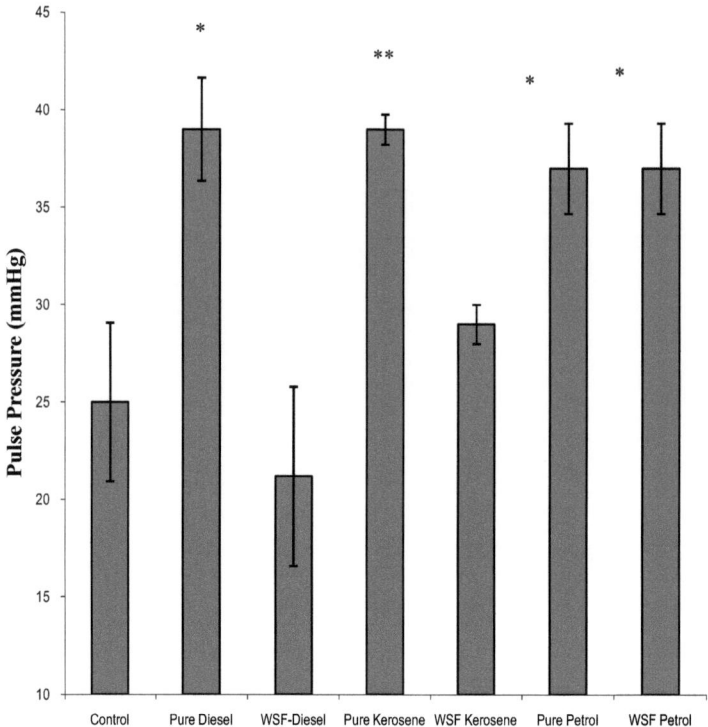

Fig.3.1.3: Bar chart showing the effect of petroleum products and their water soluble fractions on pulse pressure.
* = Significant, $P < 0.05$. ** = $P < 0.01$.

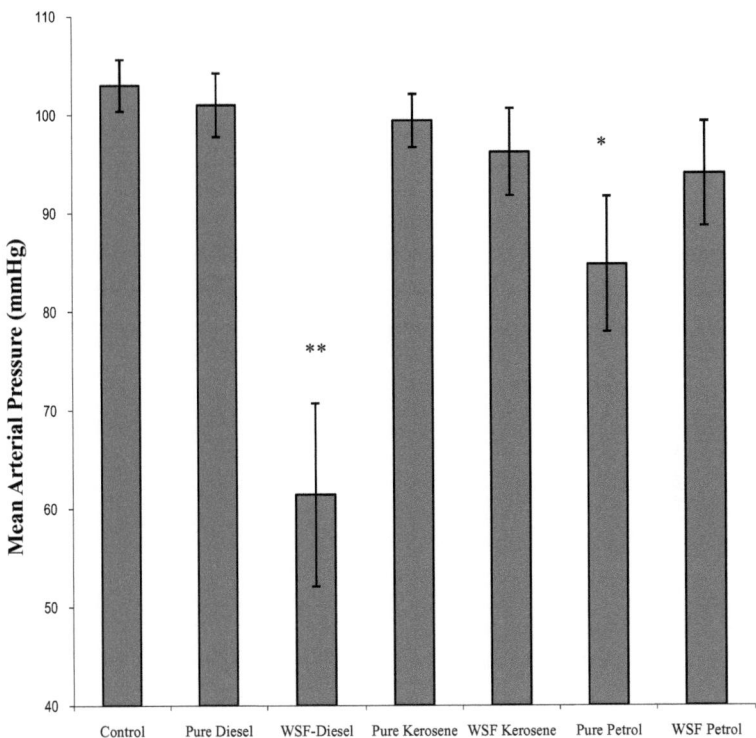

Fig.3.1.4: Bar chart showing the effect of petroleum products and their water soluble fractions on mean arterial blood pressure(MAP).
Significant * = **P** <0.05 ,   ** P < 0.01

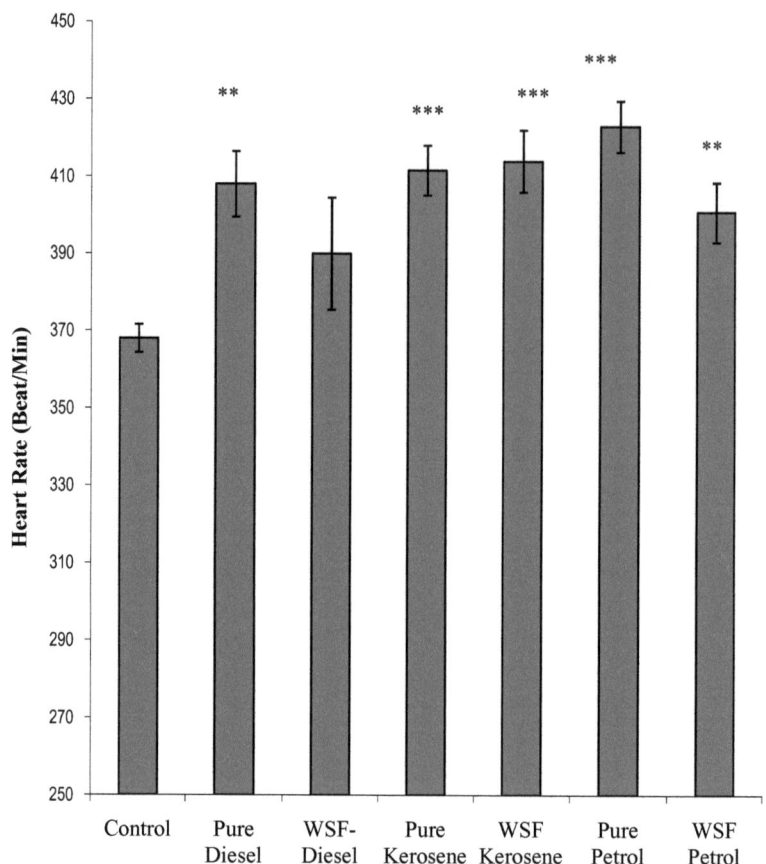

Fig.3.1.5: Bar chart Showing the effect of petroleum products and their water soluble fractions on heart rate.
Significant * = P <0.05 , ** P < 0.01, *** P < 0.001

COMPARING THE BLOOD PRESSURE AND HEART RATE OF PURE PETROLEUM FRACTIONS GROUPS WITH THEIR CORRESPONDING WATER SOLUBLE FRACTION GROUPS.

WSF-diesel had group had significant lower; systolic, diastolic, pulse pressure and mean arterial blood pressure compared to pure diesel group. But there is no significant difference in heart rate.   WSF-kerosene had significant lower pulse pressure(29 ± 1.00mmHg) P < 0.05 compared to pure diesel(37 ± 0.77mmHg). But there was no significant difference observed in; systolic blood pressure, diastolic blood pressure , mean arterial blood pressure and heart rate. There was no significant difference found in blood pressure parameters and heart rate between WSF-petrol group and pure diesel group.

34

TABLE 3.1.2: TABLE OF VALUES COMPARING THE EFFECTS OF PURE DIESEL, KEROSENE AND PETROL ON BLOOD PRESSURE AND HEART RATE WITH THEIR CORRESPONDING WATER SOLUBLE FRACTIONS.

Parameters		Pure Diesel	WSF Diesel	Pure Kerosene	WSF Kerosene	Pure Petrol	WSF Petrol
Systolic Blood Pressure (mmHg)	Mean	127	80	125.2	116	109.6	118
	SEM ±	4.8	10.96	2.92	3.85	8.13	4.10
	P.Value		*		NS		NS
Diastolic Blood Pressure (mmHg)	Mean	88	52.4	86.4	87	72.4	82
	SEM ±	2.53	9.09	2.64	4.80	6.40	6.00
	P.Value		*		NS		NS
Pulse Pressure (mmHg)	Mean	39	21.2	39	29	37	37
	SEM ±	2.65	4.59	0.77	1.00	2.32	2.32
	P.Value		*		*		NS
Mean Arterial Pressure (mmHg)	Mean	101	61.4	99.4	96.2	84.8	94
	SEM ±	3.23	9.3	2.69	4.43	6.87	5.32
	P.Value		*		NS		NS
Heart Rate (Beat/.min)	Mean	408	390	411.6	414	423	400.8
	SEM ±	8.94	14.45	6.64	8.05	6.6	7.68
	P.Value		NS		NS		NS

Significant level: *P-value <0.05, **P-value <0.01, ***P-value <0.001, NS-Non-significant P-value >0.05. SEM- Standard Error of Mean.

3.2 WEIGHT OF THE ANIMALS AND INTERNAL ORGANS

The heart weight for control was (0.78±0.04g) while treated groups were: pure diesel(0.75±0.05g), WSF-diesel(0.75±0.05g), pure kerosene(0.65±0.04g) and WSF-kerosene(0.68±0.04g) had p-value >0.05, were not significantly lower. Pure petrol(0.65±0.02g) and WSF-petrol (0.63±0.04g) were significantly lower, p<0.05.

The liver weight was higher in treated groups compared to control(9.10±0.19g). Insignificant increase was observed in WSF-diesel(9.86±0.80g), pure kerosene(9.31±0.13g) and WSF-petrol(9.81±.041g),P>0.05. SF-kerosene(9.7±0.15g) P<0.05 and pure petrol(10.95±.38g) p-value <0.01 were significantly higher. While pure diesel was significantly lower, 7.93±0.18.gWith p<0.01.

The kidney weights of treated groups showed relative lower weight except, WSF-diesel that was insignificantly higher (1.23±0.05g) P>0.05. Pure diesel(0.95±0.05g) p<0.01, pure kerosene(0.88±0.02g) p<0.001, WSF-kerosene(0.95±0.05g) P< 0.01 and pure petrol(0.93±0.07g) p<0.05 were significantly lower   but WSF-petrol-(1.10±0.07g) P>0.05 was insignificant. All compared against control(1.18±0.04g).

There was no significant difference in the weight of spleen in the treated groups compared to control(1.05±0.08g)   except pure kerosene(0.8±0.09g) that was significantly lower p-value <0.05.

TABLE 3.2.1   TABLE OF VALUES SHOWING THE EFFECTS OF PURE DIESEL, KEROSENE AND PETROL AND THEIR WATER SOLUBLE FRACTIONS ON BODY AND INTERNAL ORGANS' WEIGHT.

Parameter		Control	Pure Diesel	WSF Diesel	Pure Kerosene	WSF Kerosene	Pure Petrol	WSF Petrol
Animal Weight (g)	Mean	200	160	192	177	177	165	205
	SEM ±	3.17	3.1	8.6	3.75	3.7	7.43	11.21
	P.Value		***	NS	**	**	**	NS
Heart Weight (g)	Mean	0.78	0.75	0.75	0.65	0.68	0.65	0.63
	SEM ±	0.04	0.05	0.05	0.04	0.04	0.02	0.04
	P.Value		NS	NS	NS	NS	*	*
Liver Weight (g)	Mean	9.10	7.93	9.26	9.31	9.7	10.95	9.83
	SEM ±	0.19	0.18	0.80	0.13	0.15	0.38	0.41
	P.Value		**	NS	NS	*	**	NS
Kidney Weight (g)	Mean	1.18	0.93	1.23	0.88	0.95	0.93	1.10
	SEM ±	0.04	0.06	0.05	0.02	0.05	0.07	0.09
	P.Value		**	NS	***	**	*	NS
Spleen Weight (g)	Mean	1.05	1.00	1.28	0.8	1.1	1.08	1.24
	SEM ±	0.08	0.09	0.11	0.09	0.06	0.02	0.14
	P.Value		NS	NS	*	NS	NS	NS

Significant level: *P-value <0.05, **P-value <0.01, ***P-value <0.001, NS- Non-significant P-value >0.05. SEM- Standard Error of Mean.

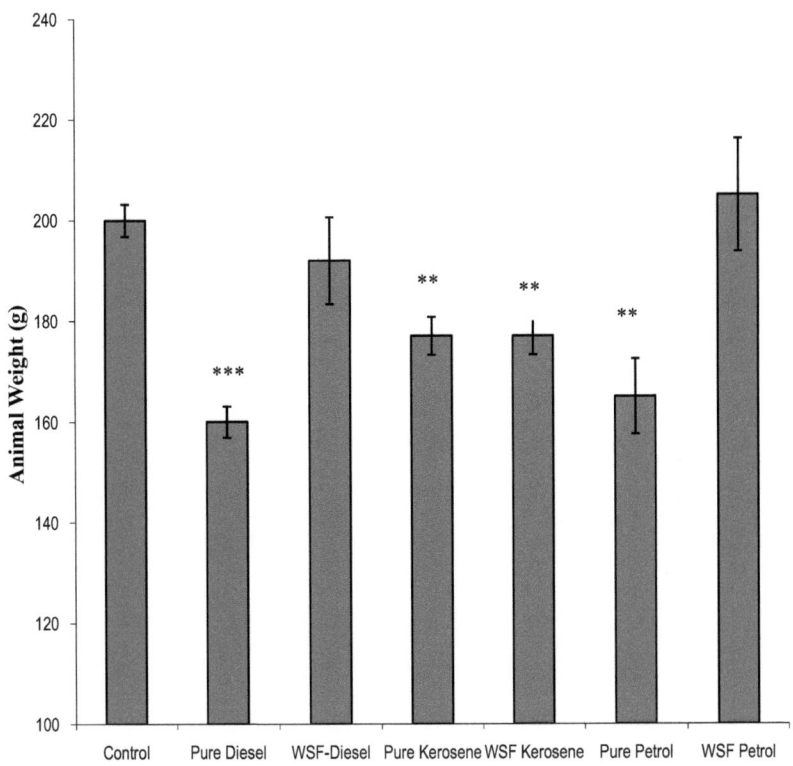

Fig.3.2.1: Bar chart showing the effect of petroleum products and their water soluble fractions on animal weight.
Significant level: *P-value <0.05, **P-value <0.01, ***P-value <0.001,

37

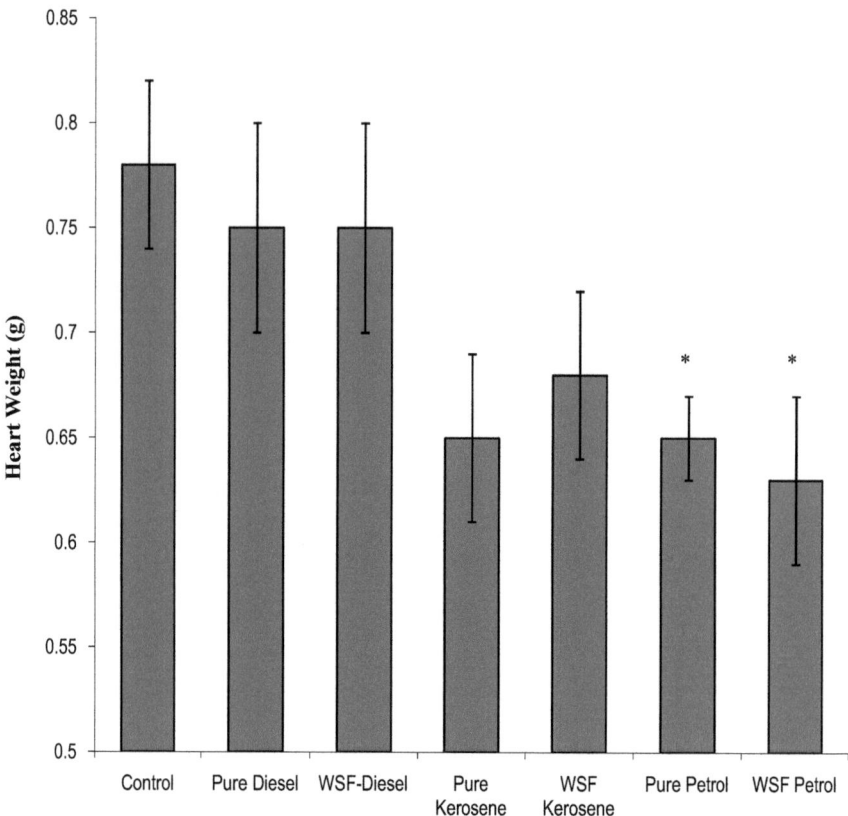

Fig.3.2.2: Bar chart showing the effect of petroleum products and their water soluble fractions on heart weight. Significant level: *P-value <0.05, **P-value <0.01, ***P-value <0.001, NS- Non-significant P-value >0.05. SEM- Standard Error of Mean.

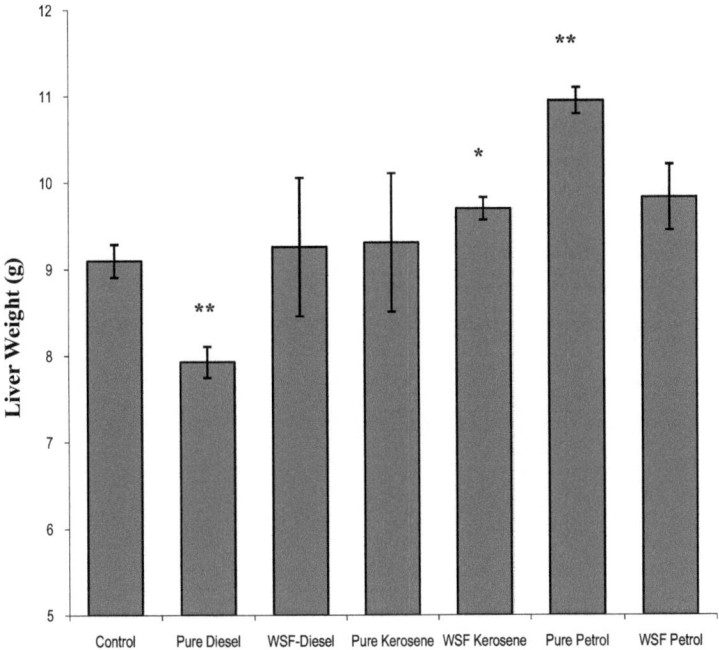

Fig.3.2.3: Bar chart showing the effect of petroleum products and their water soluble fractions on liver weight. **Significance : * P < 0.05, ** P < 0.01,**

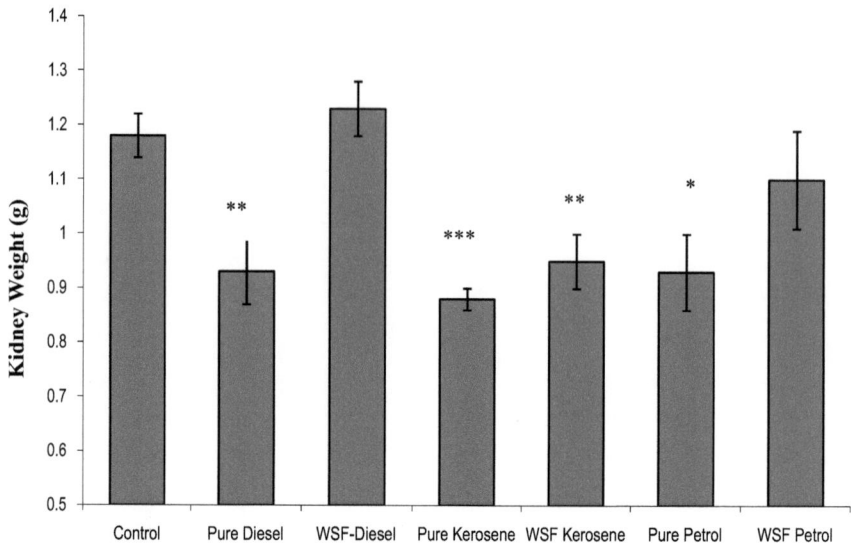

Fig. 3.2.4: Bar chart showing the effect of petroleum products and their water soluble fractions on kidney weight. Significance : * P < 0.05, ** P < 0.01, *** P < 0.001

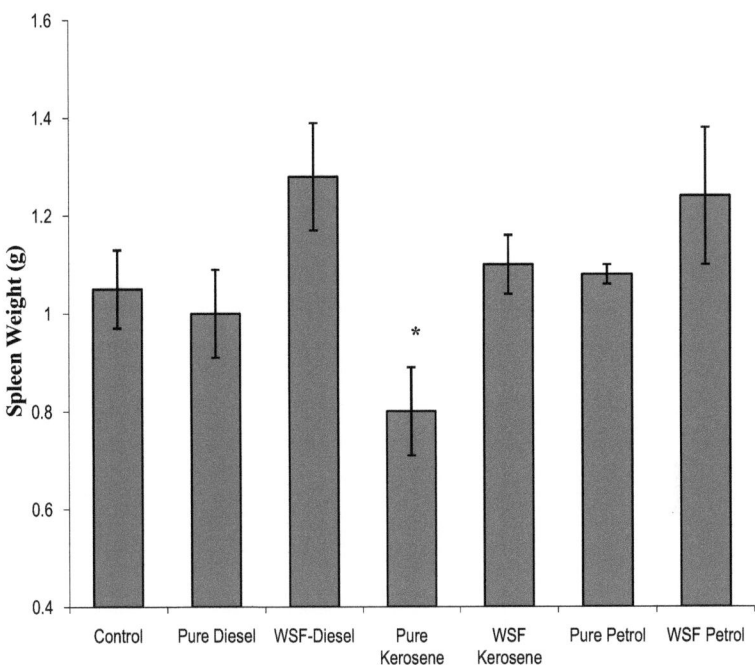

Fig. 3.2.4: Bar chart showing the effect of petroleum products and their water soluble fractions on spleen weight. Significance. * P < 0.05

3.2.1 ORGAN-BODY WEIGHT RATIO OF THE TREATED GROUPS AND CONTROL

Heart-body weight ratio was significantly higher in pure diesel group(4.08 ± 0.23) $P<0.05$ and lower in pure petrol group(3.38 ± 0.13) $P<0.05$, while others had no significant difference compared to control(3.87 ± 0.13.

Liver body-weight ratio was higher in pure kerosene(5.16 ± 0.12) and WSF-kerosene(5.47 ± 0.16) $P<0.05$, pure petrol(6.65 ± 0.10) $P<0.001$. Others were not significantly different from control(4.6 ± 0.16).

Kidney-body weight ratio was lower in pure kerosene group(4.96 ± 0.19) $P< 0.01$. Others had no significant difference compared to control(5.94 ± 0.21).

There was no significant difference in spleen-body ratio except pure petrol group(6.56 ± 0.24) $P<0.05$ compared to control(5.30 ± 0.40).

TABLE.3.2: TABLE OF VALUES SHOWING THE EFFECTS OF PURE DIESEL, KEROSENE AND PETROL AND THEIR WATER SOLUBLE FRACTIONS ON ORGAN- BODY WEIGHT RATIO.

Parameter		Control	Pure Diesel	WSF Diesel	Pure Kerosene	WSF Kerosene	Pure Petrol	WSF Petrol
Heart $x10^{-3}$	Mean	3.87	4.67	3.89	3.69	3.03	3.97	3.38
	SEM ±	0.13	0.23	0.10	0.16	0.14	0.08	0.13
	P.Value		*	NS	NS	NS	NS	*
Liver $x10^{-2}$	Mean	4.6	4.96	4.38	5.16	5.47	6.65	4.81
	SEM ±	0.14	0.19	0.26	0.12	0.16	0.10	0.14
	P.Value		NS	NS	*	*	***	NS
Kidney $x10^{-3}$	Mean	5.94	5.82	6.39	4.96	6.1	5.60	5.32
	SEM ±	0.21	0.47	0.11	0.19	0.30	0.23	0.2
	P.Value		NS	NS	**	NS	NS	NS
Spleen $x10^{-3}$	Mean	5.30	6.28	6.66	4.52	6.3	6.56	5.54
	SEM ±	0.40	0.64	0.52	0.09	0.47	0.24	0.63
	P.Value		NS	NS	NS	NS	*	NS

Significant level: *P-value <0.05, **P-value <0.01, ***P-value <0.001,   NS- Non-significance P-value >0.05. SEM- Standard Error of Mean.

3.3 THE PACKED CELL VOLUME

The comparison of the treated groups with control is shown in table3.3. The treated group had lower packed cell volume but the difference was not significant.

TABLE 3.3. TABLE OF VALUES SHOWING THE EFFECTS OF PURE DIESEL, KEROSENE AND PETROL AND THEIR WATER SOLUBLE FRACTIONS ON PACKED CELL VOLUME.

Parameter		Control	WSF Diesel	Pure kerosene	WSF Kerosene	Pure Petrol	WSF Petrol
Packed Cell Volume(%)	Mean	67	60.6	60.8	61.8	60.8	61.6
	SEM ±	2.25	2.06	2.88	1.56	2.7	1.7
	P.Value		NS	NS	NS	NS	NS

P-value: Significant level- NS- Non-significant; P >0.05; SEM- Standard Error of Mean

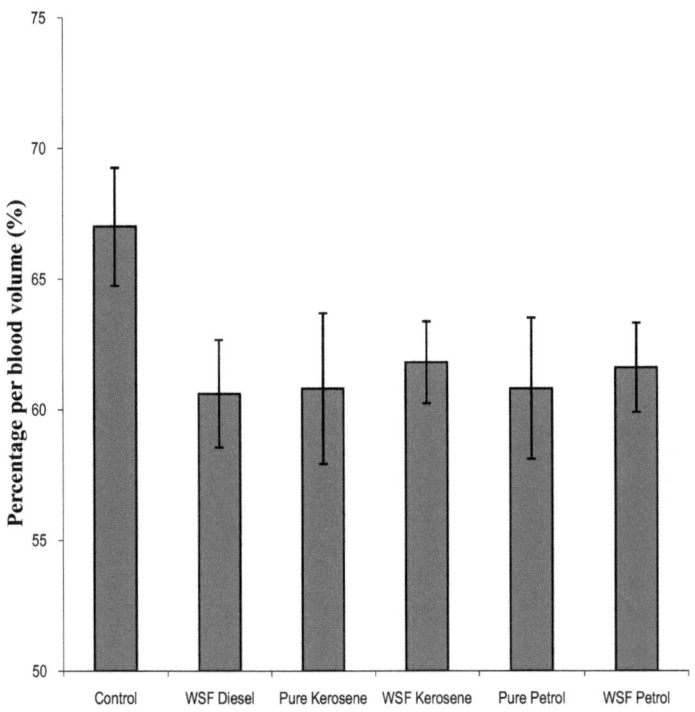

Fig 3.3. Bar chart Showing the Effect of Petroleum Products and their water Soluble Fractions on Packed cell Volume.

3.4 PLASMA LIPID PROFILE

The total cholesterol was lower in all treated groups. Pure diesel($3.5\pm$ 0.23mmol/L) $P<0.01$, Pure kerosene(3.9 ± 0.21mmol/L) $p<0.05$ and WSF-petrol(3.6 ± 0.15mmol/L) $P< 0.01$, were significantly lower. While the WSF-diesel(4.1 ± 0.31mmol/L), WSF-Kerosene(4.5 ± 0.16mmol/L) and pure petrol(4.1 ± 0.29mmol/L) were insignificant with P values higher than 0.05. Control group was 4.65 ± 0.21mmol/L.

The HDL-cholesterol was lower in all treated groups. With P-value< 0.001 in pure diesel(0.99 ± 0.07mmol/L), pure petrol(1.01 ± 0.03mmol/L) $P<0.001$ and WSF-Petrol(1.25 ± 0.5mmol/L) $P<0.01$. While WSF-diesel(1.38 ± 0.11mmol/L), pure kerosene(1.38 ± 0.07) and WSF-kerosene(1.55 ± 0.06mmol/L) were not significant when compared with control(1.60 ± 0.07mmol/L).

The LDL-cholesterol was lower in all the treated groups: WSF-diesel(2.3 ± 0.17mmol/L) and WSF-kerosene(2.5 ± 0.10mmol/L) had P-value > 0.05 were not significant. While pure diesel(1.95 ± 0.13mmol/L) $P<0.01$, pure

43

kerosene(1.96±0.10) P<0.01, pure petrol(19±0.07mmol/L) P<0.05 and WSF petrol(1.90±0.08mmol/L) P<0.01 were significantly lower.

The triglycerides was higher in treated groups than control group(0.90±0.04mmol/L) except pure petrol(0.88±0.03mmol/L)P>0.05 was insignificantly lower. The pure diesel(1.24±0.08mmol/L), pure kerosene(1.22±0.07mmol/L), WSF-Kerosene(1.06±0.03mmol/L) and WSF-petrol(1.06±0.05mmol/L) were significantly higher with P- value < 0.05. The WSF-diesel(1.01± 0.08mmol/L) was not significant P>0.05.

TABLE 3.4. TABLE OF VALUES SHOWING THE EFFECTS OF PURE DIESEL, KEROSENE AND PETROL AND THEIR WATER SOLUBLE FRACTIONS ON PLASMA LIPID PROFILE.

Parameters		Control	Pure Diesel	WSF Diesel	Pure Kerosene	WSF Kerosene	Pure Petrol	WSF Petrol
Total Cholesterol (mmol/L)	Mean	4.65	3.5	4.1	3.9	4.5	4.1	3.6
	SEM ±	0.21	0.23	0.31	0.21	0.16	0.29	0.15
	P.Value		**	NS	*	NS	NS	**
HDL-Cholesterol (mmol/L)	Mean	1.60	0.99	1.38	1.38	1.55	1.01	1.25
	SEM ±	0.07	0.07	0.11	0.07	0.06	0.03	0.05
	P.Value		***	NS	NS	NS	***	**
LDL Cholesterol (mmol/L)	Mean	2.61	1.95	2.3	1.96	2.5	2.19	1.90
	SEM ±	0.14	0.13	0.17	0.10	0.10	0.07	0.08
	P.Value		**	NS	**	NS	*	**
Triglycerides (mmol/L)	Mean	0.90	1.24	1.01	1.22	1.06	0.88	1.06
	SEM ±	0.04	0.08	0.08	0.07	0.03	0.03	0.05
	P.Value		*	NS	*	*	NS	*

Significant level: *P-value <0.05, **P-value <0.01, ***P-value <0.001, NS-Non-significant P-value >0.05. SEM- Standard Error of Mean.

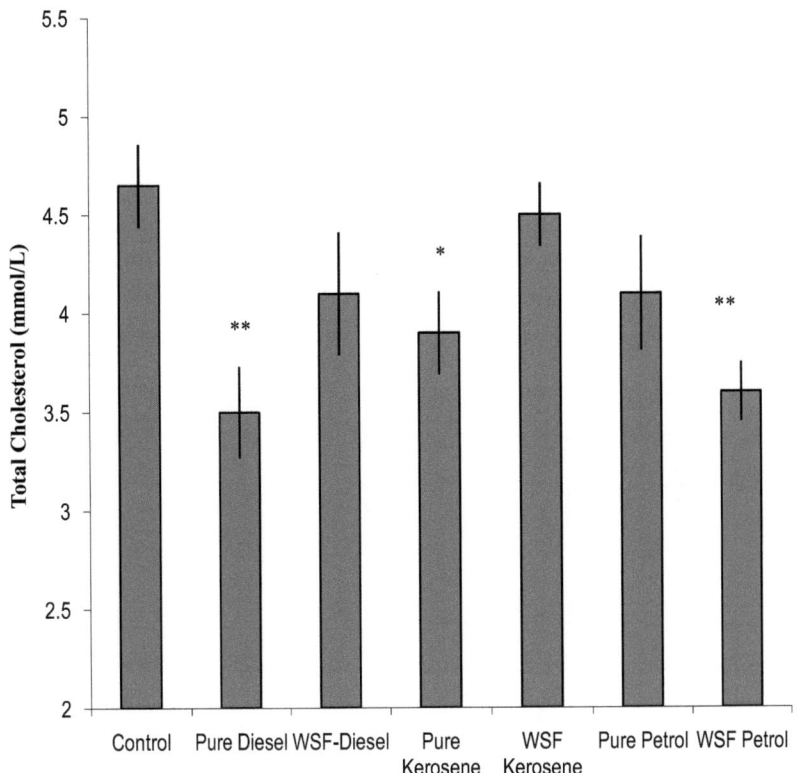

Figure 3.4.1   Bar showing the Effect of Petroleum Products and their Water Soluble Fractions on plasma Total Cholesterol
Significant level: *P-value <0.05, **P-value

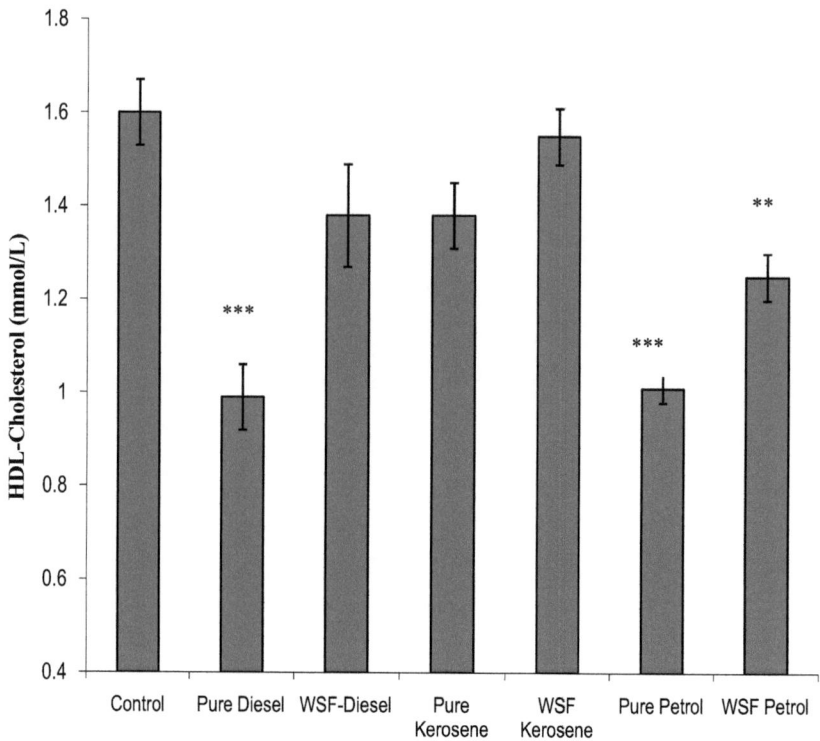

Figure 3.4.2 Bar showing the Effect of Petroleum Products and their Water Soluble Fractions on HDL-Cholesterol
Significant level: *P-value <0.05, **P-value <0.01, ***P-value <0.001,

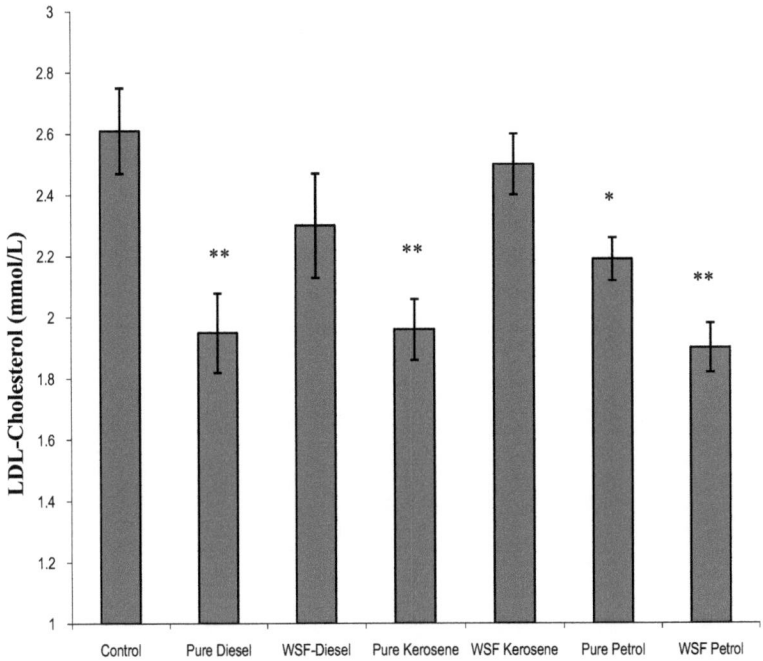

Figure 3.4.3   Bar chart showing the Effect of Petroleum Products and their Water Soluble Fractions on plasma LDL-Cholesterol
Significant level: *P-value <0.05, **P-value <0.01

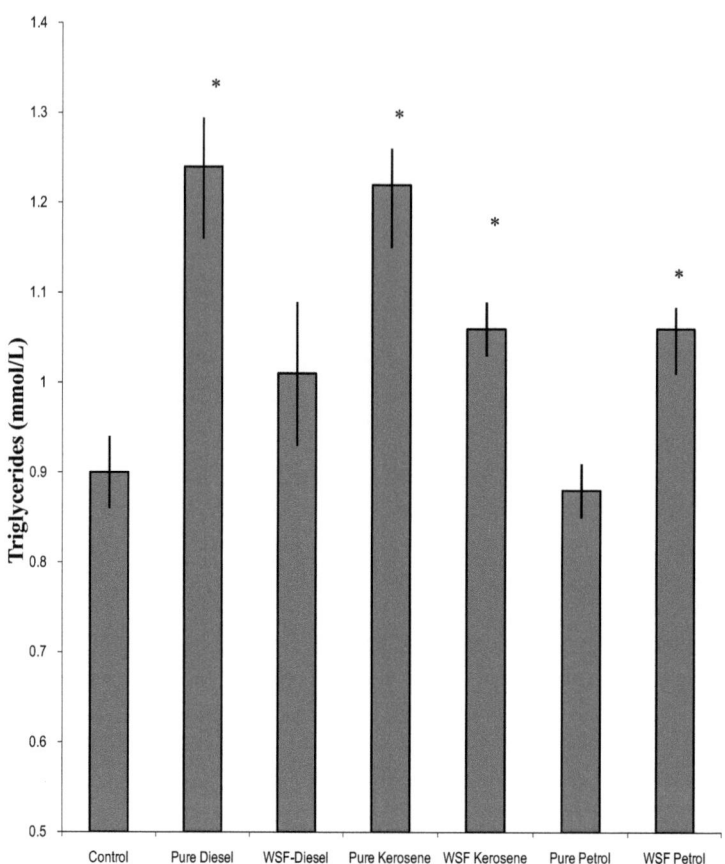

Figure 3.4.4 Bar showing the Effect of Petroleum Products and their Water Soluble Fractions on plasma Triglycerides
Significant: * P < 0.05

COMPARING THE EFFECT OF PURE PETROLEUM FRACTIONS ON PLASMA LIPID PROFILE WITH THEIR CORRESPONDING WATER SOLUBLE FRACTIONS.

WSF-diesel of diesel had higher HDL-cholesterol (1.38±0.11mmom/l) P<0.05 compared to pure diesel(0.99±0.06mmol/L), while there was no significant difference found in total cholesterol, LDL-cholesterol and triglyceride. WSF-kerosene had higher LDL-cholesterol(2.52±0.10mmol/L) P< 0.01, compared to pure kerosene(1.97±0.10mmol/L). There was no significant difference in others.

WSF-petrol had higher HDL-cholesterol(1.25±0.05mmol/L) P<0.01 and triglycerides(1.06±0.046mmol/L) P <0.05 , compared to pure petrol (1.01±0.05 mmol/L) and (0.87±0.03mmol/L) respectively. LDL-cholesterol was lower in WSF-petrol(1.91±0.08 mmol/L) P <0.05, compared to control(2.19±0.07 mmol/L). There was no significant difference in total cholesterol level between pure and corresponding WSF treated groups.

TABLE 3.4.2: TABLE OF VALUES SHOWING THE COMPARISON OF THE EFFECTS OF PURE DIESEL, KEROSENE AND PETROL WITH THEIR CORRESPONDING WATER SOLUBLE FRACTIONS ON PLASMA LIPID PROFILE.

Parameter		Pure Diesel	WSF Diesel	Pure Kerosene	WSF Kerosene	Pure Petrol	WSF Petrol
Total Cholesterol (mmol/L)	Mean	3.5	4.12	3.92	4.51	4.08	3.62
	SEM ±	0.23	0.31	0.21	0.16	0.29	0.15
	P.Value		NS		NS		NS
HDL-Cholesterol (mmol/L)	Mean	0.99	1.38	1.38	1.54	1.01	1.25
	SEM ±	0.06	0.11	0.07	0.06	0.03	0.05
	P.Value		*		NS		***
LDL Cholesterol (mmol/L)	Mean	1.95	2.32	1.97	2.52	2.19	1.91
	SEM ±	0.12	0.18	0.10	0.10	0.07	0.08
	P.Value		NS		**		*
Triglycerides (mmol/L)	Mean	1.19	1.02	1.18	1.06	0.87	1.06
	SEM ±	0.09	0.08	0.08	0.03	0.03	0.05
	P.Value		NS		NS		*

Significant level: *P-value <0.05, **P-value <0.01, NS: Non-significant P-value >0.05. SEM: Standard Error of Mean.

CHAPTER FOUR
DISCUSSION
A major problem facing dwellers in the Niger Delta environment of Nigeria and other areas where there are petroleum installations like pipeline and refineries is related to pollution by petroleum products. This pollution often results in diffused chronic exposure or massive acute exposure as occur in blow outs and vandalism. These sub-lethal concentrations may not necessarily lead to outright mortality but may have significant effects which can lead to physiological stress and dysfunctions (Omoregie, 1998).

4.1 BLOOD PRESSURE AND HEART RATE
In this study, the systolic blood pressure of the treated groups showed no significant difference compared to control except the group treated with water soluble fraction of diesel which was significantly lower than the control. The diastolic blood pressure was lower in all treated groups compared to control. The pulse pressure was higher in all treated groups, but only insignificantly lower in water soluble fraction of diesel treated group. The mean arterial blood pressure (MAP) was higher in control than treated groups. The heart rate was higher in all the treated groups compared to control(table3.1). Pure diesel fraction had increased blood pressure parameters relative to its corresponding water soluble fractions(table3.1.2).

The increase heart rate observed in the treated groups might be due to lower blood volume resulted from anaemia induced by hydrocarbon (Sudiakov, 1992). The heart rate increased in order to maintain normal perfusion since the stroke volume is expected to be lower. The reduced heart size observed may decrease the pumping efficiency of the heart. The wider pulse pressure observed could be due to decreased vascular compliance. Noa and Illnait, (1987), stated that exposure to kerosene aerosol or to smoke product from kerosene caused aortic plaques with fibrous tissue, collagen and elastic fibres that interspersed within the smooth muscle cells resembled those seen in arteriosclerosis. ASTDR, (1995), reported that breathing fuel vapour for period as short as one hour may cause increase in blood pressure. Chronic human exposure to petrol fuel could be a risk factor in the aetiology of hypertension. Xylene is an hydrocarbon component of petrol and it causes depression, fatigue, headache, anxiety, feeling of drunkenness and sleep disorder. All these are potent pressor stimuli (Akintonwa and Oladele, 2000).

Hinshaw et al., (1966), studied the effects of chlorinated hydrocarbon on the cardiovascular system in dogs and reported a marked increase in venous return within 30 min, significant fell in total peripheral resistance that remain low, no observed changed in pulmonary vascular resistance , there was increase in blood catecholamine. The chlorinated hydrocarbon was found to be toxic to the left ventricle; left heart failure demonstrated by elevated left atrial pressure regularly occurred.

4.2. WEIGHTS OF INTERNAL ORGANS AND ANIMAL
All the treated groups had significantly lower mean weight compared to control(table 3.2), except the water soluble fraction of petrol group which had an

insignificant increase in mean body weight. The lower body weight might not unrelated to changes in the metabolic pathway induced by hydrocarbons. Ben-David et al., (2001) submitted that the ingestion of petroleum caused reduction in blood glucose. This may shift the demand for metabolic substrate to lipid and protein. Berepubo et al., (1994), also stated that a relatively short exposure to crude oil led to the inhibition of growth in weaned rabbit.. Wong et al (1994) reported similar observation in juvenile pink salmon (Oncorhynchs gorbusvcha). These reports supports the findings of this study, this is due to metabolic stress induced by hydrocarbons.

All the treated groups had higher liver weight compared to control, except the pure diesel treated group which had significantly lower liver weight. The lower liver weight found in this group might correspond to absolute lower mean body weight of this group compared to the control group. Kerosene and petrol had higher liver-body weight ratio. Poons et al.,(1997) reported that male rats given 200mg/kg/day (benzothiophene) for 21 days by gavage study showed relative increase in liver weights. Brady eta.(19990), reported that gasoline treatment alter microsomal monoxygenase activities in rats . Poons and colleagues also reported increase in serum enzymes like gamma-glutamyltransferase and hepatic alaline hydroxylase. The increase in hepatic activities might be responsible for increase in weight in the treated group. Dede and Kagbo (2001) stated that diesel is hepatotoxic by causing narrowing of sinuses and severe hepatocellular necrosis.

All the treated groups has relatively lower heart weight compare to the control. A significant decrease in weight was seen in pure petrol treated and water soluble fraction of petrol treated group. Diesel group had increased heart-body weight ratio. Mehlman and Legator(1991), stated that 1,3 butadiene cause heart hemagiosarcomas.

All the treated groups had significantly lower mean kidney weight compare to control except water soluble fraction of diesel and water soluble fraction of petrol treated groups which showed insignificant increase in kidney weight. Pure kerosene group had decreased kidney-body weight ratio. Poon et al.(1997), reported increase in kidney weight and 4.5 fold increase in urine volume in rats treated with benzothiophene (sulphur containing hetero-cyclic hydrocarbons). USDHH, (1993), also reported that hydrocarbons has kidney and liver effects. Dede and kagbo showed diesel is nephrotoxic by distrupting tubular mechanism and latter causing necrosis of tubular cells. Mehlma, (1992), reported a significant increase in kidney tumour in rats treated with gasoline. There is no significant difference in the spleen of treated groups compared to control except the pure kerosene group that had significant lower mean weight. Pure petrol had higher spleen-body weight ratio.

4.3 PACKED CELL VOLUME

The result of this study showed that there is decrease in packed cell volume in treated groups though without any significance(table3.4). But the works of others has demonstrated significant decrease in PCV. Linear reduction in haemoglobin, packed cell volume, platelets and erythrocytes count was observed in crude oil treated rabbit (Ovuru and Ekweozor, 2003). Similar toxic components like chlorinated hydrocarbons exert the same effects on blood cell profile (Mastsumuta, 1975). In the same vein, the toxic components in petroleum products change the blood chemistry and induce anaemia and interfered with platelet production in animals (Sudakov, 1992).

The study of Okoro and colleagues (2006) also corroborates the toxicity of hydrocarbons on bone marrow: they observed a significant fall in haemoglobin, packed cell volume, red blood cell and white blood cell in human study exposed to petroleum fumes for a number of years. This supported the assertion that benzene, xylene and lead are activated in bone marrow. The cytotoxic effects are mediated through disturbance in DNA function (Rabble *et al*, 1996). The report of this study supports the view of previous studies.

4.4 PLASMA LIPID PROFILE

In this present study, effects of some petroleum products and their water soluble fractions on plasma lipids profile was analysed. It was found out that, the control had higher total cholesterol, HDL-cholesterol and LDL-cholesterol, while the triglycerides was higher in the treated groups except the pure petrol treated group (Table 3.4). But the observed higher LDL-cholesterol and lower triglycerides contradicts the findings of earlier authors like Achuba, (2005). Who discovered reciprocal relationship between HDL-cholesterol and LDL-cholesterol in the plasma of rabbit fed with crude petroleum contaminated di*et*

During the past decades, a vast amount of evidence has confirmed that lipid and lipoprotein abnormalities play a major role in the pathogenesis and progression of arteriosclerosis and cardiovascular diseases (Ginsberg, 1994). These chronic degenerative disorders have become a growing health problem worldwide. In African populations, dyslipidemia as a risk factor for cardiovascular disease and increasing incident of death due to cardiovascular disease in both urbanized and underdeveloped rural countries have been reported (Van der Sande *et al*., 2001).

Ben- David *et al,*. (2001) submitted that the ingestion of petroleum products caused reduction in blood glucose, this may shift demand for metabolic substrate to lipid, thus explaining the significant lower in triglycerides contrary to the report of this study. HDL and LDL cholesterols are two of the four main groups of plasma lipoproteins that are involved in lipid metabolism and the exchange of cholesterol, cholesterol ester and triglyceride between tissues. (Sviridiv,1999).

Numerous population studies have shown an inverse correlation between plasma HDL levels and risk of cardiovascular disease, implying that factors associated with HDL protect against atherosclerosis. Some of these factors appear to be anti-oxidant, anti-inflammatory effects which may obviate processes that initiate atherogenesis (Oram and Lawn, 2001). Epidemiological study has also shown that elevated concentration of total cholesterol and LDL-cholesterol in the blood are powerful factor for coronary heart disease (Lawn, 1999). Most extra-hepatic tissues although have a high requirement for cholesterol have low activity of the cholesterol biosynthetic pathway. These cholesterol requirements are supplied by LDL which is internalised by receptor-mediated endocystosis. Through lecithins: HDL cholesterol also regulates the exchange of proteins and lipids between various lipoproteins, HDL provides the protein component required to activate lipoprotein which releases fatty acids that can be oxidised by the B-oxidation pathway to release energy, most importantly HDL-cholesterol can inhibit oxidation of LDL-cholesterol as well as the artherogenic effects of oxidized LDL-cholesterol by virtue of its antioxidant property (Sviridiv, 1999; Ademuyiwa *et al.*, 2005).

Dyslipidemia is known to cause endothelia dysfunction, a dysfunctional endothelium will express impaired nitric oxide production activity as well as alteration in endothelium I and endothelium A and B receptors expression (Ruben *et al*, 2006). Dyslipidemia has been shown to be related to both early and late stages of chronic renal failure (Crook *et al*, 2003). According to Ruben *et al.*, (2006), it is also co-risk factor for hypertension along with obesity and diabetes. The oxidative modification of the LDL-cholesterol, causes macrophages to take up LDL particles through a receptor-independent pathway and increasing atherogenicity of LDL-cholesterol particles (Austin *et al*, 1990).

4.5 CONCLUSION

Oral administration of petroleum products in this study showed no consistent significant difference in plasma lipid profile of the control and treated groups. It had no significant effect on systolic blood pressure. It lowered diastolic blood pressure and increased pulse pressure. It significantly increased heart rate. It insignificantly reduces packed cell volume while respiratory rate was insignificantly increased. It reduced body weight, heart weight, kidney weight and increased liver weight. It also increased liver-body weight ratio, spleen-body weight ratio and reduced kidney–body weight ratio.

4.6 RECOMMENDATION

More work needs to be done on the effect of petroleum fractions on the parameters examined in this study.

REFERENCES.

Acuba F.I., Osakwe S.A. (2003). Petroleum induced free radical toxicity in African catfish (charas garie premis). *Fish Physiology and Biochemistry. 29:97-103*

Achuba F.I. (2005). Effects of vitamin C and E intake on blood lipid concentration, lipid peroxidation, superoxide dismitase and catalase activities in rabbits fed petroleum contaminated di*et Parkistan J. of Nutrition. 4(5):330-335.*

ACGIH (1997). Threshold limit values and biological exposure indices for 1989-1990. American Conference of Governmental Industrial Hygienist, Cincinati, Ohio.

Ademuyiwa O., Ugbaja R.N., Idumebor F. and Adebawo O. (2005). Plasma lipid profiles and risk of cardiovascular diseases in occupational lead exposure in Abeokuta, Nigeria. *Lipid in Health and Disease. 4:19.*

Adonaylo V. N. and Oteiza P. (1999). Pb^{+2} promotes lipid oxidation and alterations in membrane physical properties. *Toxicology. 123:19-32*

Ailman T. J., Godsland I. F., farren B., Crook D., Wong H.J. and Scott J. (1997). Defects of insulin action on fatty acid and carbohydrate metabolism familial combined hyper-lipidemia. *Arteriosclerosis, Thrombosis and Vascular Biology. 17:745-54.*

Al-Mahroos F., Al-Roon K. and Mckeique P.M. (2000). Relation of high blood pressure to glucose intolerance, plasma lipid and education status in Arabian Gulf population. *International Journal of Epidemiology. 29:71*-6.

Allain C.C., Poon C. S. G., Richmond W and Fu P.C. (1974). *Clinical Chemistry. 20:470.*

Amadi A., Dickson A. A. and Maat (1993). Remediation of oil polluted soils. Effect of organic and inorganic supplementation on the performance of maize (Zeamay). *Water, air and soil pollution. 66:59-76.*

Amaozie O. I. and Onwumah I. N. (2001). Toxic effect of Bonny light crude oil on rats after ingestion of contaminated di*et. Nigeria Journal of Biochemistry Molecular Biology. (proc. Suppl) 16:1035-1085.*

Anguilar-Salinas C.A., Ohaiz G., Valles V., Torres J. M. R., Perez F. J. G., Rull J. A., Roajas R., Fronco A. and Sepulveda J. (2001). High prevalence of low HDL-cholesterol concentration and mixed hyperlipidemia in a Mexican nationwide survey. *Journal of Lipid Research. 42:1298-1307.*

Anigbogu C. N. and Adigun S. A(1996). Blood pressure, Heart rate and autonomic reflexes in plasmodium Berghei malaria infection. *Nigeria Qt. Journal of Hospital Medicine.6(1):47-51.*

Anigbogu C. N. and Adigun S. A(1987). Effects of chloroquine on Cardiovascular response to carotid occlusion in rats. *Nigeria Journal of Physiological Science 4; 75.*

Astrand I., Kilbom A. and Oltrun P. (1975). Exposure to white sprout. I concentration in alveolar, air and blood during rest and exercise. *Scandinavian Journal of Work, Environment and Health. 1:15-30.*

ATSDB, (1995). Agency for toxic substances and disease registry. Toxicological profile for fuel oils. Atlanta, G.A. US Department of Health and Human Services, Public Health Services.

Austin I, King M., Vranizan K., Krauss R. (1990). Artherogenic lipoprotein phenotype. *Circulation. 82:495-8.*

Baden S. G. (1982). Oxygen consumption rate of shrimp exposed to crude oil extract. *Marine Pollution Bulletin. 13(7):230-233.*

Badiman J. I., Badiman L and Fuester U. (1990). Regression of artherosclerotic lesion by HDL plasma fraction in cholesterol-fed rabbit. *Journal of Clinical Investigation. 85:1234-1241.*

Ben-David M., Duffy L. K., and Bowyer R. T. (2001). Bio-maker responses in river otters experimentally exposed oil contamination. *Journal Wildlife Diseases. 37:489-508.*

Berepubo N. A., Johnson N. C and Sese B. T. (1994). Growth potentials and organ weight of weaner rabbit exposed to crude oil contaminated feed. *International Journal Animal Science. 9:73-76.*

Bohlen P. Schlingerr U. P. and Lauppi E. (1973). Uptake and distribution of hexane in tissue. *Toxicology Applied Pharmacology. 25:242.*

Braddy J. F., Xiao F., Gapac M. J., Ming M.S. and Yang S.C. (1990). Alteration of rat liver microsomal monooxygenase activities. *Archives of Toxicology. 64(8):677-79.*

Browing E. (1965). Toxicity and metabolism of industrial solvents, Amsetedam, lauda, New York, Elsevier Publishing Company.

Cairney B. (2005). Petrol in the brain. *American Environmental Journal. pp: 1.*

Cheesbrough, M. (2002): PCV and Red Cell Indices, Haematological Tests in: Cheesbrough, M. (Ed.). District Laboratory Practice in Tropical Countries Part2, Pp. 310 - 314.

Clayton G. D. and Clayton F. E.. Patty's industrial hygiene and toxicology. Volume IIB. 3rd revised ed. John Willey and Sons, New York, 1981).

Crook E. D., Thallapureddy A., Migdal S., Flock J. M., Gren E. L., Salaudeen A., Tucker J. K. and Taylor (2003). Abnormalities and renal diseases: Is dyslipidemia a predator of progression of renal disease? *American Journal Medical Science. 325(6):340-348.*

Dede E. B. and Kagbo H. D. (2001). Investigation of acute toxicology effects of diesel fuel on rats (rattus rattus) using histopathological method. Journal of *Applied Science and Environmental Management. 5(1)_:83-84.*

Dede E. B and Kagbo H. D. (2005). Aqua-toxocological effects of water soluble fraction of diesel (WSF) fuel oil on O. niloticus fingerlings. *Journal of Applied Science Environmental Management. S(1):93-96.*

Egan B. M. (2003). Insulin resistance and the sympathetic nervous system. *Hypertension Research. SS: 247-254.*

Egborge A. B. M. (1991). Industrialization and heavy metal pollution in Warri River. 32nd inaugural lecture. University of Benin, Benin City. Nigeria.

Ehrhardt M. and Heineman J. (1975). Hydrocarbon in blue messels from the Kiel Bight. *Environmental Pollution. 9: 265-281.*

EPA, (2003). Environmental protection Agency: The toxic effect of environmental pollution.

Floodgate G. D. (1972). Microbiology degradation of oil. Marine *Pollution Bulletin. 3:41-43.*

Fourmas D. W. and Hine C. H. (1958). Neurotoxicity of selected hydrocarbons. *Arch. Ind. Health. 18:9-15.*

Gaisberg H. N. (1994). Lipoprotein metabolism and its relationship to atherosclerosis. *Medical Clinic of North America. 78:1-20.*

Garcia M. M., Gonzalez A. R. and Casaco P.A. (1988). Biochemical mechanism in the effects of kerosene on airways of experimental animals. *Allergologia Imunopathologia. (Madr.) 16(5):363-7.*

Gerade H. W. (1963). Toxicological studies on hydrocarbons IX. The aspiration hazard and toxicity of hydrocarbons and hydrocarbon mixtures. *Archives Environmental Health. 6:329-41.*

Gerade H. W. (1959). Toxicological studies on hydrocarbons. V. Kerosene. *Toxicology and Applied Pharmacology. 1:462-474.*

Gloriosos N., Troffa C., Filighedu F., Dettori F., Soro A., Pargagha P.P., Collatina S. and Pahor M. (1999). Effects of the 3-hydroxy.3-methylglutaryl (HMG) – co-enzyme A (CoA) reductase inhibitor on blood pressure on patient with essential hypertension and primary hypercholesterolemia. *Hypertension. 34:1281-1286.*

Gotto a. m.(1988). Lipoprotein metabolism and the etiology of hyperlipidemia. *Hospital Practice. 23:sppl. 1-4*

Gupta K. and Mehoratra N. K. (1990). Mouse skin ornithinase decarboxylase induction and timuor promotion by cyclo-hexane. *Conc. Lett. 15:227-233.*

Haines J. R. and Alexandar M. (1974). Microbial degradation of high molecular weight alkanes. *Applied Microbiology. 28(6):1084-1085.*

Hinshaw L.B., Solomon L.A., Reins D.A., Fiorica V and Emerson T.E. (1966). Effects of the insecticide endrin on the cardiovascular system of the dog. *Journal of Pharmacology and Experimental Therapeutics. Vol. 153, Issue 2, 225-236.*

Hoegstedt B., Gullberg B., Mark V.E., Mitelmon F and Skerving S. (1981). Micronuclei and chromosome aberration in bone marrow cells; and lymphocytes of human exposed mainly to petroleum vapour. *Heraditas. 94:179-87.*

Hoekstra W. G. and Philips P. H. (1963). Effects of topically applied mineral and fractions on the skin of guinea pigs. *Invest. Dermatol. 40(2):79-88.*

IARC (1989). Intenational Agency for the Research on Cancer. Occupational exposures in petroleum fuels. IARC monograph on the evaluation of carcinogenic risk to lungs.

ICEP. (1993). International Cholesterol Education Programme. Summary of the National Cholesterol Education Programme (NCEP). Expert panel on detection evaluation and treatment of high blood cholesterol in adults. *Journal of American Medical Association. 269:3015-3025.*

Ichihara K., Kusunase E. and Kusunase M. (1969). Microsomal hydroxylation of decane. *Biochimica et Biophysica ACTA. 176:713-719.*

IPCS,(1982).International Programme on Chemical Safety. Enviromental Health criteria 20 .Selected Petroleum Products. World Health Organisation, Geneva ,1982.

Jacob P. G. and Al-Meizaini (1995). Marine plant of Arabian Gulf and Effects of oil pollution. *Mahasagar. 23:83-101.*

Jee S. H., Wang J. D., Sun C. C. and Chao Y. F. (1986). Prevalence of probable kerosene dermatoses among ball-bearing factory workers. *Scandinavian Journal of Work and Environmental Health. 12:61-65.*

Kennicutt M.C., Sweet S.F (1992). Hydrocarbon contamination on the Antarctic Peninsula III. The Bahia Paraiso two years after the spill. *Marine Pollution Bulletin. 25(9-12):303-306.*

Khan M. A. Q., Al-Gharis S. M and Al-Maris (1975). Petroleum hydrocarbon from fish from the Arabian Gulf. *Archives of Environmental Contamination and Toxicology. 29(4):517-522.*

Kiihnhold W. W. (1980). Some aspects of the impact of aquatic oil pollution on fishery resources. FAO/UNDP. South China Sea Fisheries Development and Coordinating Programme. *Manilla, Phillipines. P1-26.*

Koschier F.J. (1999). Toxicity of middle distillate from dermal exposure. *Drug and Chemical Toxicology. 22:155-64.*

Krechmann K. H., Robert L. G. and Staab R.J. (1998b). Inhalation. Inahalation multigeneration reproductive study with cyclohexane in rats. *Toxicological Sciences. 42:1-5.*

Lipovskij S. M. (1978). The serotonin content in the tissue of uterus and particulars on its contracting activities under the influence of petroleum solvents vapours. *Gig. Tr. Prof. Zabol. Nop. 7:37-40.*

Lipovskij S. M., Tomaeva L. V., Varfolomence D. I., Fedoseev J. G. and Kargoanova E. U. (1979). The accumulation of petroleum solvents on the tissue and organs of pregnant women.. *Gig. Tr. Prof. Zabol.*

Law M. R. (1999). Lower heart disease risk with cholesterol reduction: evidence from observational studies and clinical trials. *European Heart Journal. Suppl. 1:53-58.*

Mason B. (1966). The concentration of minor elements in biogenic deposits. Principles of geochemistry, 3rd ed. New York. John Wiley & Sons Inc. pp 241-243.

Matsmura F. (1975). Energy of insecticides into animal systems in toxzicology of insecticides. *Pler, Press, New York, USA. Pp. 165-179.*

Mehlman M. A. (1992). Dangerous and cancer-causing properties of products and chemicals in the oil refinning and petrochemical industry-carcinogenicity of gasoline. *Environmental Research. 59(1): 238-49.*

Miles L., Fless G., Levin E., Scami A. and Plow E. (1989). A potential basis for the thrombotic risk associated with lipoprotein A. *Nature. 339:301-303.*

Miyagaki H. (1967). Electrophysiological studies on the peripheral neurotoxicity of n-hexane. *Japan Journal of Industrial Health. 9:12-23*

Mraz J.E., Gabva H and Vilkova (1998). 1,2 and 1,4 cyclo-hexandiol, major urinary metabolites and iron makers of exposure to cychlohexane, cyclohexanone and cyclohexanol in human.

Noa M. and Illail J. (1987). Changes in the aorta of guinea pigs exposed to kerosene. *Acta Morphologica Hungarica. 35 (1-2):59-69.*

Mofer J. R., Tepel M., Kehiel B., Wierwile S., Walter M., Seedorf U., Zidek W., Assman G. (1997). Low density lipoprotein inhibits the sodium/hydrogen antiport in human platelets. A novel mechanism enhancing platelet activity in hypercholesterolemia. *Circulation. 95:1370-77.*

Nomiyama K. and Nomiyama H (1974). Retention uptake and excretion or organic solvents in man. *Int. Arch. Arbeitsmed. 32:75-91.*

Novikov k. L., kolodina L. N., Lipovskij S. Mand Badalova L.(1979). Lactation parameters in female workers of the chemical(rubber) industry. *Grig. Tr. Prof. Zabol. No. 2pp45-48.*

Okoro A. M., Ani E. J., Ibu J. O.and Akpogomeh B. A. (2006). Effects of petroleum products inhalation on some heamatological indices of fuel attendants in Calabar Metropolis, Nigeria. *Physiological Society of Nigeria. 21:(1-2) pp 71-75*

Omoregie E. (1998): Changes haematology of Tilapia (oreochromis noloticus trewoves) under the effect of crude oil. *Acta Hydrobiologica. 40:289-292.*

Oram J.F. and Law R.M. (2001). ABCA 1: The gatekeeper for eliminating excess tissue cholesterol. *Journal of lipid Research. 42:1170-1179*

Ovuru S.S. and Ekweozor I.K.E. (2004). Haematological changes associated with crude oil ingestion in experimental rabbitrs. *African Journal of Biotechnology. 3 (16):346-348.*

Petroleum Handbook (1966). London Shell International Petroleum Company Limited.

Poon R., Davis H., Lecavalier P., Liteplo R., Yagnimas A., Chin I and Bihi C. (1997). Effects of benzothiophene on male rats following short term oral exposure. *Journal of Toxicology. And Environmental . Health. 50(1):53-56.*

Quinlan G. F., Halliwell B. Moorehouse C. P. and Gutteridge M. C> and (1981). Action of lead (II) and Aluminium ions on iron stimulated lipid peroxidation in liposomes, erythrocytes and rat liver microsomal fractions. *Biochemica et Biophysica Acta. 962: 196-200*

Rabble G.K. and Wong O. (1996). Intracellular leukemia mortality by cell type in petroleum workers with potential exposure to benzene. *Environmental Health Perspectives. 104:138-1392.*

Riihimaki U., Pfafeli P., Savolainnen k. (1979). Kinetics of m-xylene in man .General features of absorption , distribution biotransformation and excretion in repetitive exposure. *Scandinavian Journal of Work and Environmental Health .5:217-231*

Riihimaki U. (1979). Percutaneous absorption N-xylene from a iso-xylene and isomethyl alcohol on man. *Scandinavian Journal of Work and Environmental Health. S. 143-150.*

Ritchie G., Still k., Ross J. 3rd, Beckedal M., Bobb A. and Arfsten d. (2003). Biological and Health effects of exposure to kerosene based -jet fuel and performance additives. *Journal of Toxicology and Environmental Health part-B Critical Review. 6:357-451.*

Ruben O. H., Sesso D. H., Ma J., Burning J. F., Stampfer M. J. and Gaziomo J. M. (2006). Dyslipidemia and the risk of incidence of hypertension in men. *Hypertension.* 47:45-50.

Sabo D. J. and Stageman J. J. (1977). Some metabolic effects of petroleum hydrocarbons in marine fish. In: Physiological response of marine biota to pollutants, Verberg F. J., Cobaresse A., Thirbirg F.P., Boemberg W. (eds). *Academic Press New York, oo. 279-287.*

Schanplein R. J., Blank I. H., (1971). Permeability of the skin. *Physiological Reviews. 51:702-747.*

Shen B. J., Todaro J. F., Niawa R., McCaffery J. M., Spiro A. 3rd and Word K.D. (2003). Are metabolic risk factor one unified syndrome? Modeling the structure of metabolic syndrome X. *American Journal Epidemiology. 157:701-711.*

Sinmers M. H. (1964). Petroleum asphalt inhalation by mice. *Archives of Environmental Health. 9(6):723-724.*

Spencer P. S., Bischoff M. C. and Schaumburg H. H. (1978). On the specific molecular configuration of neurotoxic aliphatic hexacarbon compound causing peripheral distal neuropathy. *Toxicology and Applied Pharmacology. 44:17-28.*

Sumammur P.k. and Susianti W.(1979). Skin and other affections in gasoline and diesel oil pump workers. *Indones J. Ind. Hyg. Occup. Health,11-12:20-22*

Steinberg D. M. and Witzun J. (1990). Lipoprotein and atherosclerosis. Current Concepts. *Journal of American Medical Association. 264:3047-3052.*

Sudakov K. V. (1992). Stress postulate: Analysis from the position of general theory of functional system. *Pathophysiological and Experimental Therapeutics. 4:86-93.*

Sviridiv D. (1999). Intracellular cholesterol trafficking. *Histology Histopathology. 14:305-319*

Symth H. F. and Smith H. F. (1928). Inhalation experiment with certain lacquer solvents. *J. Ind. Hig. 10:261-271.*

Tagami H. and Ogino A.(1973). Kerosene dermatitis; Factors affecting skin irritability to kerosene. *Dermatological,146:123-131*

Tietz N. W. Textbook of clinical chemistry, 3rd Ed. C. A. Burtis, E. R. Ashwood, and W. B. Sander (1999)pp: 809-57.

USEPA (1997). U.S Enviromental Protection Agency. Integrated Risk Information System (IRIS). On current National Center for Environment Assessment, Office Research and Development, Washington, DC 1997.

USDHHS (1993). U.S Department of Health and Human Services Hazardous substance data bank (HSDB, online Database). National Toxicology Information Program, National Library of Medicine, Bethsida. M.D.

USDHHS (1993). US Department of Health and human Services (1993). Registry of toxic effects of chemical substances (RTEFCS, online Database). Toxicology Information Program, National Library of Medicine, Bethsida.

Wang S. Y., Lum J. L., Carls M. G., and Rice S.D. (1994). The relationship between growth and total nucleic acid in juvenile pink salmon (oncorhynchus porhusha) Fed crude and contaminated Fed. *Canadian Journal of Fisheries and aquatic Sciences. 50:996-1007.*

Wang C.C.(1961). Acute gasoline intoxixation. *Archives Environmental Health. 2:714-716*

Williams R. T. (1959). Detoxification mechanism 2nd ed. New York, John Willey & Sons Inc.

Yuasa J., Kishi R., Eguchi T., Harabuchi I., Kawa T. l, Ikeda M., Sugimoto R., Matsumoto H., Miyake H. (1996). Investigation on neurotoxicity of occupational exposure to cyclohexane: a neurophysiological study. *Occupational and Environmental Medicine. 53:174-17.*

Zingmark P.A. and Rappe C. (1977). On the formulation of N-nitrosodi-ethanolamine in a grinding concentrate after storage. *Ambio:237-238*

APPENDIX I

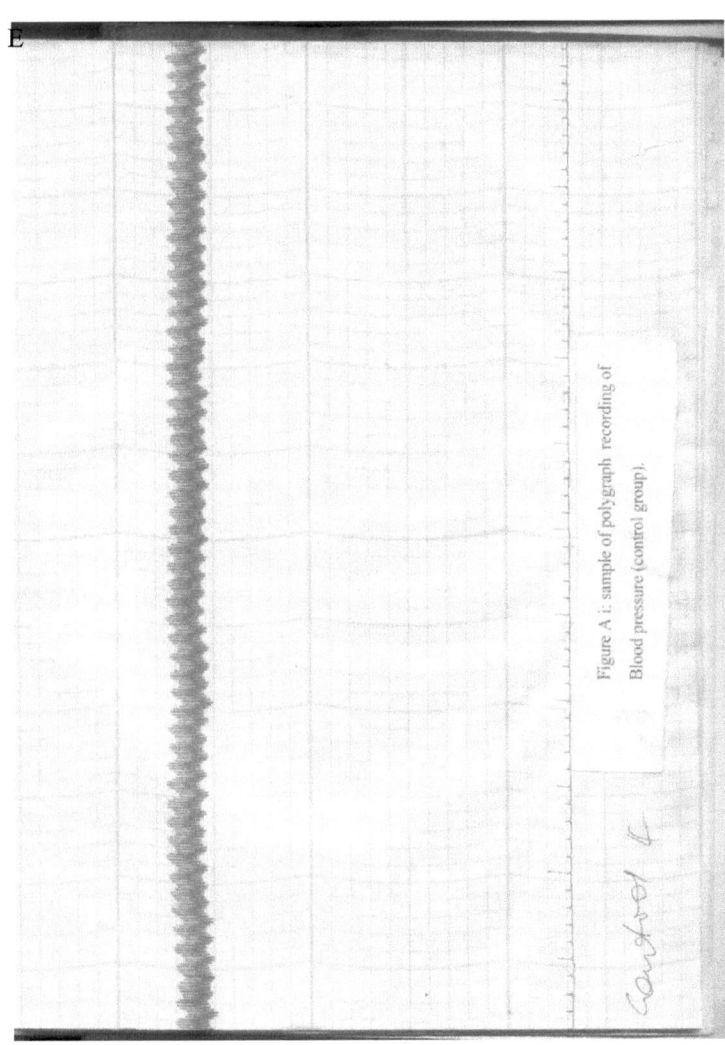

Figure A i: sample of polygraph recording of
Blood pressure (control group).

APPENDIX II

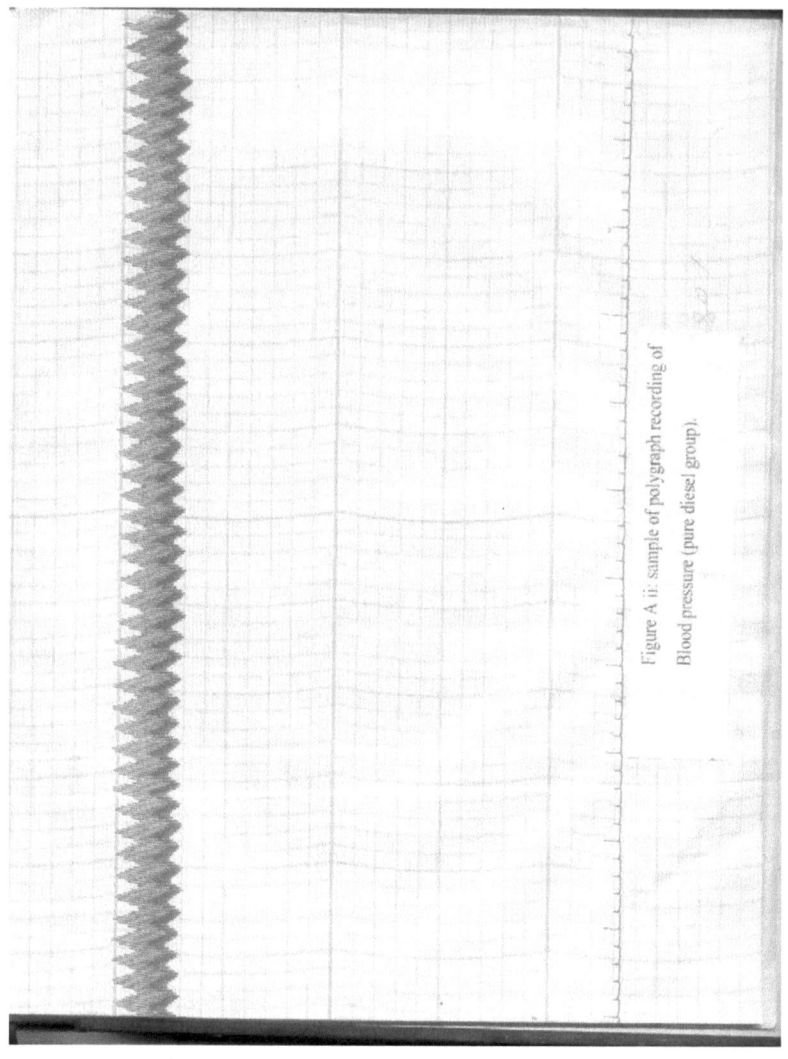

Figure A ii: sample of polygraph recording of Blood pressure (pure diesel group).

APPENDIX III

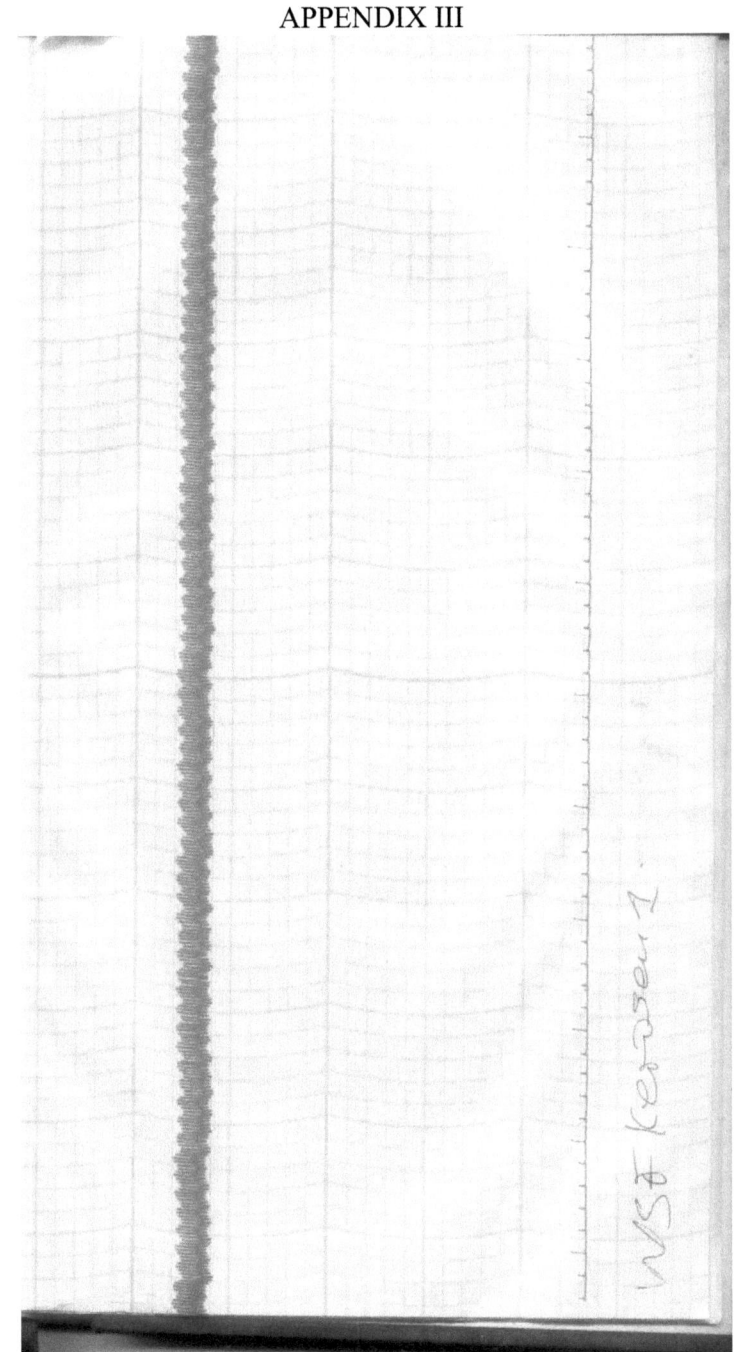

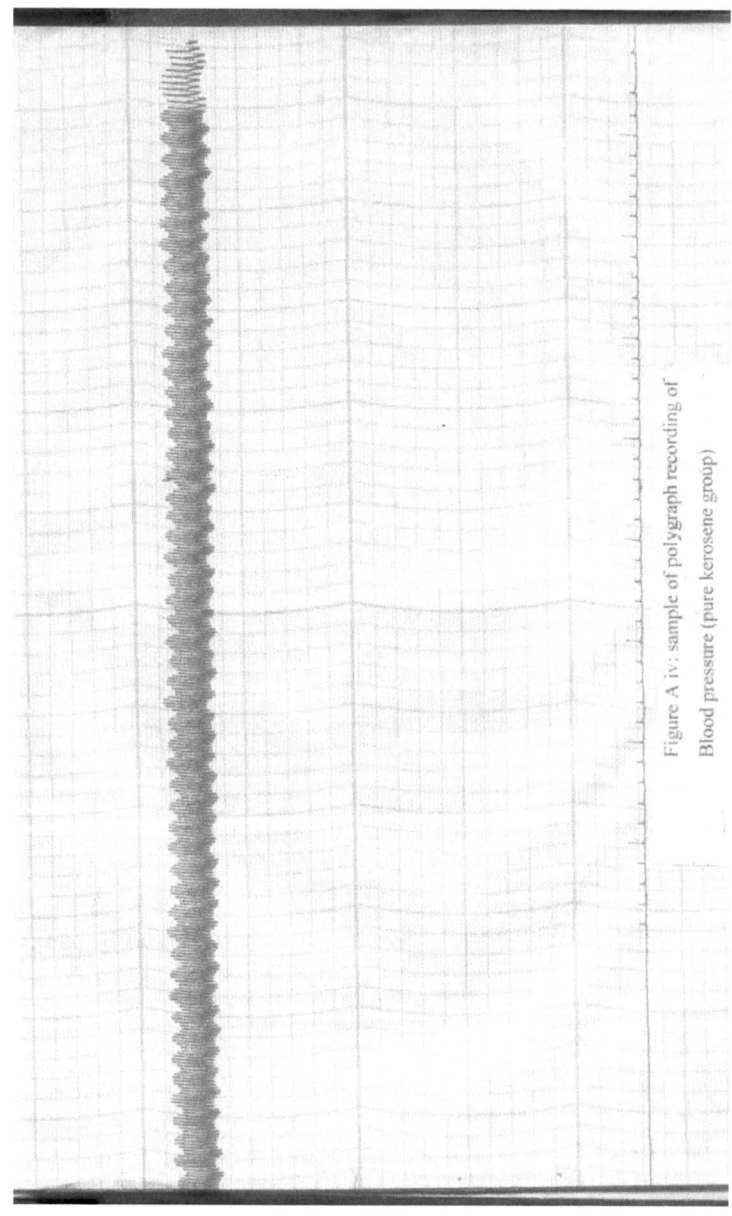

Figure A iv: sample of polygraph recording of
Blood pressure (pure kerosene group)

APPENDIX V

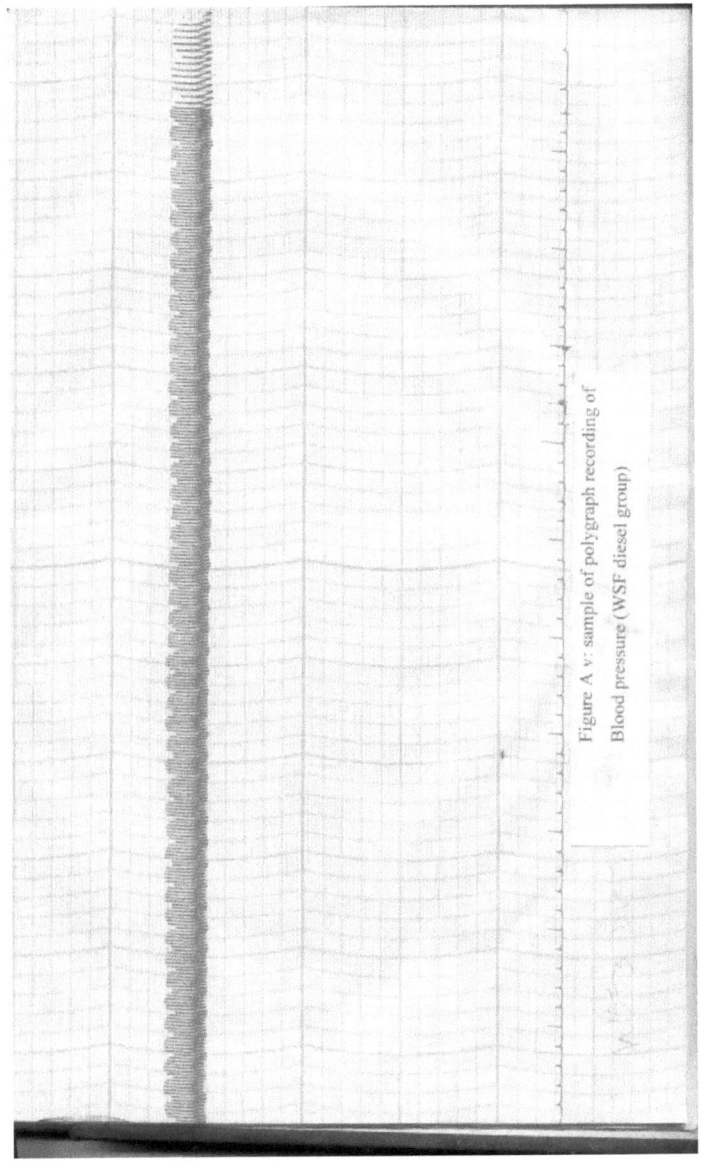

Figure A v: sample of polygraph recording of
Blood pressure (WSF diesel group)

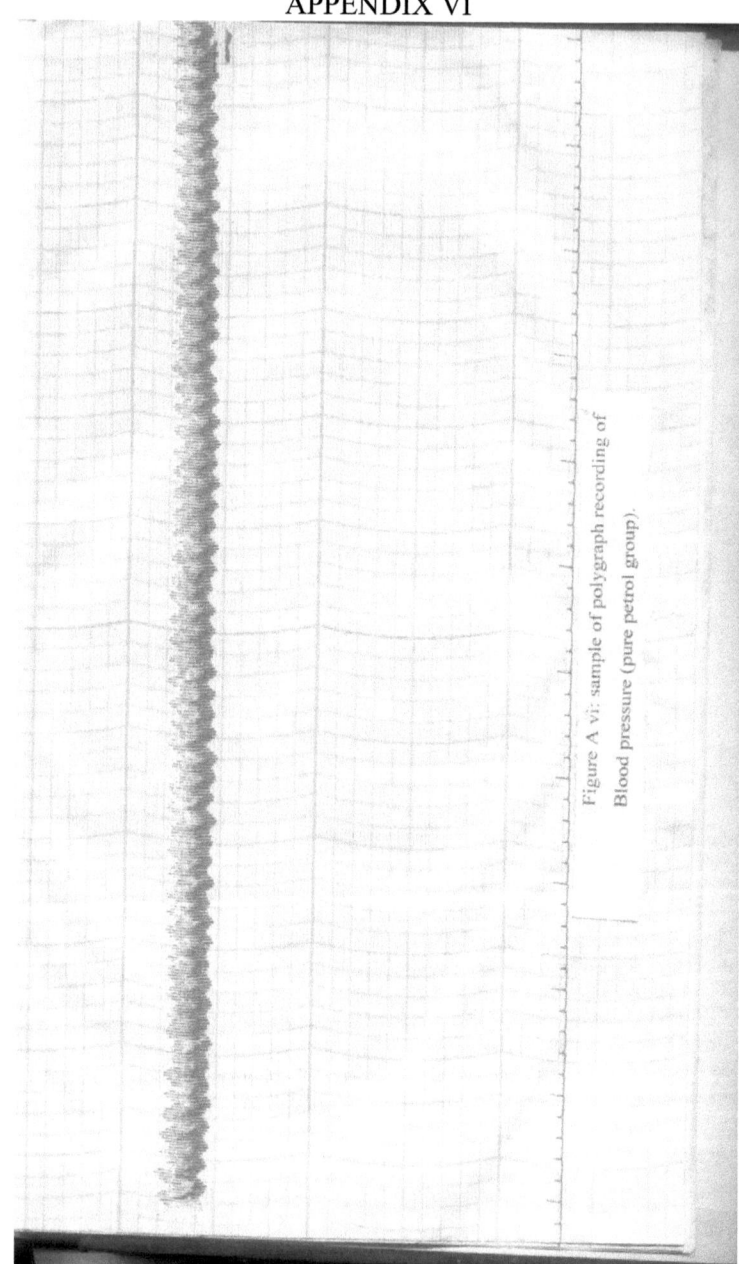

Figure A vi: sample of polygraph recording of Blood pressure (pure petrol group).

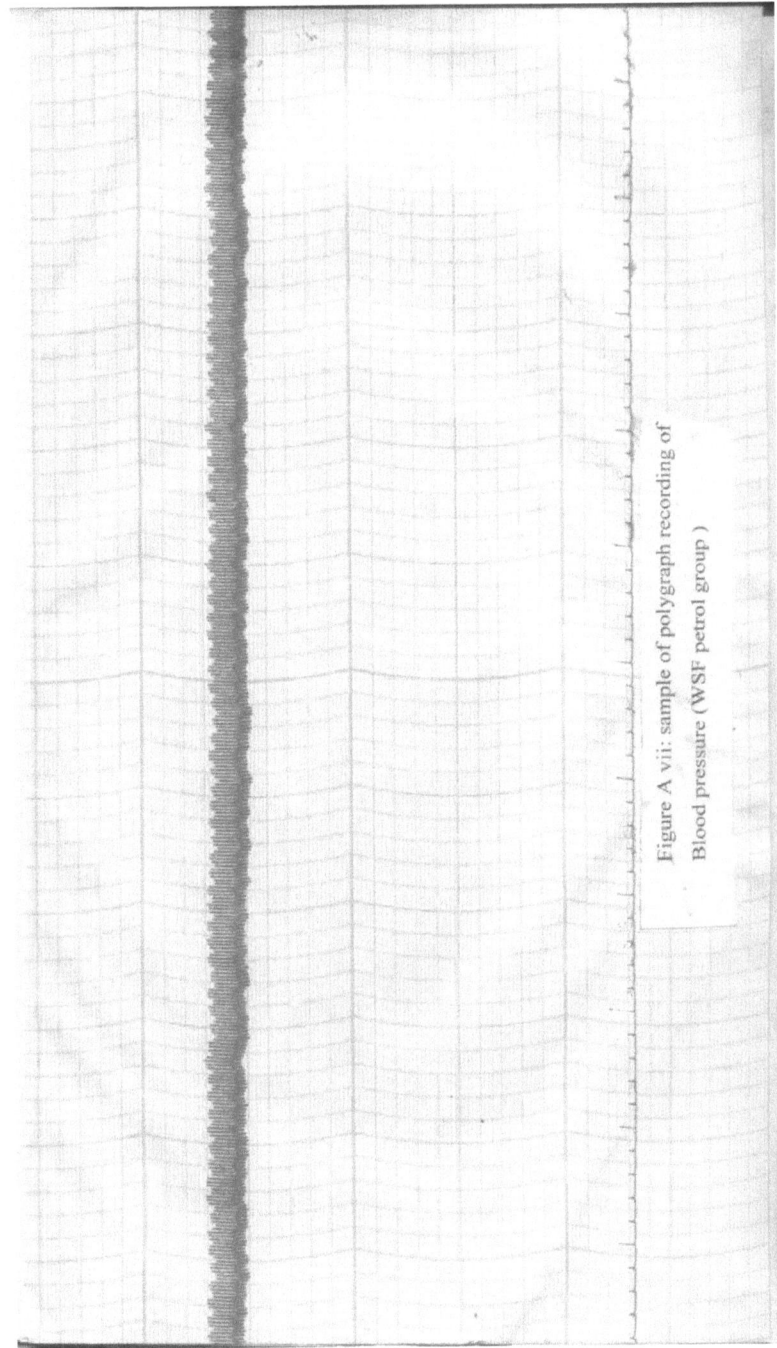

Figure A vii: sample of polygraph recording of Blood pressure (WSF petrol group)

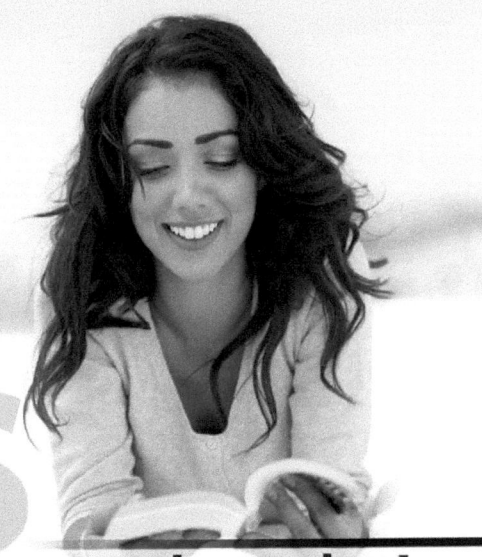
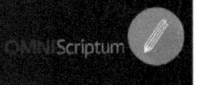

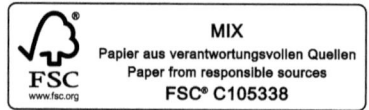